Unmasking Autism: The Cross-Cultural

Revolution in Adult Assessment

Dr. Sai Achuthan & Dr. Dave Barker

BlueRoseONE.com
Stories Matter

BLUEROSE PUBLISHERS UK Ltd.
London

This book is primarily published and distributed in Great Britain and is also available in other global marketplaces.

ISBN: 978-93-7139-352-2

Designed and distributed by **BlueRoseONE.com** with global reach. Printing and fulfilment are managed through international distribution networks, ensuring availability based on order locations.

For publishing inquiries, visit **www.BlueRoseONE.com**

BlueRose Publishers UK Ltd,
Unit 3, 6-7 St Mary at Hill, London
+44 7386286323

First Edition: October 2025

Dedication

To all the autistic adults who have waited too long for recognition and understanding.

To the clinicians who strive to see beyond stereotypes and truly understand the individuals they assess.

And to our families, who have supported us through the countless hours of clinical work and writing that made this book possible.

Acknowledgments

We extend our deepest gratitude to the many individuals who have contributed to the development of this comprehensive training resource and our understanding of autism across cultures.

First and foremost, we thank the countless autistic individuals and their families who have shared their experiences with us over the years. Your insights, challenges, and triumphs have shaped our clinical understanding and driven our commitment to improving assessment practices.

We are profoundly grateful to our families for their unwavering support:

Mrs Usha Devi Padmanabhan and Mrs Haema Priya Achuthan, whose wisdom and encouragement have been instrumental in shaping our perspectives on neurodiversity and cultural sensitivity.

Laxmi Kutty Padmanabhan, for her invaluable insights into cross-cultural understanding.

Mr Colin Barker and Ms Dionne Barker, for their steadfast support and understanding throughout the long hours dedicated to clinical practice and writing.

Miss Kelly Turner and Mr Brian Turner, for their perspectives on lived experience and their commitment to autism awareness.

Ms Amanda Coates, for her exceptional support that kept this project on track.

We also acknowledge our esteemed colleagues who have contributed their expertise and insights:

Dr Uthish Sreedaran, for his pioneering work in culturally sensitive assessment approaches and his mentorship in navigating complex diagnostic challenges.

Dr Joanna Farrow, for her expertise in female autism presentations and her dedication to addressing gender disparities in diagnosis.

Psychiatry UK – one of the largest private online neurodevelopment assessment platforms providing exceptional guidance

Insight Diagnostics Global – Academic training for neurodevelopmental understanding alongside assessment.

Dr Nnamdi Chi-Nwankwo, for his valuable contributions to understanding autism in African communities and his advocacy for equitable assessment practices.

Dr Sunday Udensi, for his insights into neurodevelopmental assessment across diverse populations and his commitment to reducing diagnostic disparities.

Dr Karl Solangbalansay, for his innovative approaches to autism assessment in Southeast Asian communities and his work in developing culturally adapted assessment tools.

We thank the many institutions and organizations that have supported our work, including the NHS trusts and Independent Sector / Private Sector where we have practiced, the universities that have hosted our research, and the autism organizations that have facilitated our engagement with the autistic community.

Special recognition goes to the participants in our training programs over the years, whose questions, challenges, and feedback have helped refine and improve the content presented in this book.

Finally, we acknowledge the broader autism community—researchers, clinicians, advocates, and most importantly, autistic individuals themselves—who continue to advance our understanding of autism as a fundamental aspect of human neurodiversity.

While we have strived to create a comprehensive and culturally sensitive resource, we recognize that our understanding continues to evolve. Any limitations or oversights in this work remain our responsibility alone.

Dr. Sai Achuthan

Dr. Dave Barker

May 2025

Intended Audience

This comprehensive training program is specifically designed for:

- Psychiatrists and Psychiatric Trainees seeking to develop specialized expertise in adult autism assessment beyond standard psychiatric training
- Clinical Psychologists working in neurodevelopmental, mental health, or adult assessment services
- Specialist Autism Assessment Teams requiring advanced training in complex presentations
- Mental Health Professionals regularly encountering undiagnosed autism in their practice
- Neuropsychologists expanding their practice to include comprehensive autism evaluation
- Speech and Language Therapists specializing in adult communication disorders
- Occupational Therapists working with sensory processing and adult neurodevelopmental conditions
- Clinical Nurse Specialists in autism or adult mental health settings
- Medical Directors establishing or improving autism assessment services
- Academic Researchers studying adult autism presentation and assessment
- Clinical Leads responsible for service development and quality improvement in autism pathways
- Professionals Conducting Remote Assessments who need to understand the critical nuances of online vs. in-person evaluation

This training is particularly valuable for professionals working in diverse settings who encounter culturally complex presentations and those seeking to improve identification of autism in historically underdiagnosed populations, including women, culturally diverse communities, and adults with co-occurring mental health conditions.

Participants should have foundational clinical knowledge and experience working with adult populations. While focused on the unique challenges of adult assessment, this program provides the advanced skills necessary to transform diagnostic practice and recognize autism presentations frequently missed by standard approaches.

Contents

Introduction

In a world where autism assessment remains trapped in outdated paradigms and cultural blind spots, this comprehensive training program shatters conventional wisdom and transforms clinical practice. "**Unmasking Autism: A Revolutionary Cross-Cultural Approach to Adult Assessment**" challenges everything you thought you knew about identifying autism in adults especially those who don't fit the textbook mould, while providing the most evidence-based, practical framework available today.

Drawing from the controversial yet groundbreaking clinical insights of Dr. Sai Achuthan and Dr. Dave Barker, this training confronts the uncomfortable truth that most clinicians miss autism in adults—particularly in women, culturally diverse populations, and those with co-occurring conditions. Their combined decades of cross-continental expertise reveal how Western-centric assessment models fail countless individuals and how our understanding of autism must evolve beyond simplistic stereotypes.

This is not just another professional development course on autism. It's a radical rethinking of neurodevelopmental assessment that will both challenge and support you:

WHAT YOU WILL LEARN

Challenging the Status Quo:

- Why traditional assessment tools consistently fail adults, especially women and those from non-Western cultures
- How clinician bias leads to devastating misdiagnosis and missed diagnosis
- Why online assessment works brilliantly for some but dangerously fails others
- The uncomfortable truth about how mental health conditions can mask autism—and how most clinicians get it wrong

Supporting Clinical Excellence:

- 50 meticulously detailed chapters covering every aspect of adult autism assessment
- Step-by-step guidance through complex differential diagnosis with extensive case examples
- Evidence-based approaches supported by over 100 recent research citations
- Practical frameworks that can be implemented immediately in clinical practice

Whether you're a psychiatrist, psychologist, or specialist clinician, this training will transform your practice. One that is **culturally informed, clinically rigorous, and deeply human.** Those who embrace this revolutionary approach will identify autism others miss, provide life-changing diagnoses to those previously overlooked, and elevate their clinical practice to new heights of cultural competence and diagnostic precision.

The future of autism assessment isn't found in simply applying childhood models to adults—it requires the courage to challenge established practices and embrace a truly dimensional, culturally-informed understanding of neurodevelopmental diversity. This training provides exactly that, combining controversial insights with supportive frameworks that will change not just how you assess autism, but how you understand it.

CHAPTER 1

Introduction to ASD Assessment

Welcome to this comprehensive training on **Autism Spectrum Disorder (ASD)** assessment in adults. For psychiatrists and trainees working within the UK healthcare system, understanding how to effectively assess for ASD in adult populations is becoming an increasingly essential clinical skill.

This training aims to equip you with the knowledge, skills, and confidence to conduct thorough, evidence-based assessments that adhere to UK clinical standards and guidelines.

The landscape of autism diagnosis has evolved dramatically over recent decades. Historically, autism was primarily conceptualized as a childhood condition, with diagnosis focused almost exclusively on children presenting with more obvious or 'classic' traits. Today, we know better. Many individuals—particularly those without intellectual disabilities, those with strong compensatory strategies, and women—often reach adulthood without appropriate identification and diagnosis. This has created what some researchers term a "lost generation" of adults with undiagnosed autism, many of whom have struggled without understanding the neurobiological basis of their difficulties.

In the UK, adult autism diagnosis has gained significant recognition following the **Autism Act 2009**, the first disability-specific legislation in England. This Act mandated the creation of an adult autism strategy and statutory guidance, emphasizing the importance of diagnostic pathways for adults. The **NICE Clinical Guideline 142** (updated in 2021) provides our framework for autism assessment in adults, and this training is aligned with these guidelines.

Why is proper assessment so crucial?

First and foremost, accurate diagnosis provides an explanation and framework for understanding lifelong difficulties that many adults with undiagnosed autism have experienced. This understanding alone can be transformative, reducing self-blame and confusion while providing a neurobiological context for differences in social communication, sensory processing, and cognitive style. For many, diagnosis offers more than clarity: it offers **relief, self-understanding, and validation**.

Clinically, a formal diagnosis unlocks access to essential services and protections, including:

- **Workplace accommodations** under the Equality Act 2010
- **Specialist support and therapy services**
- **Eligibility for disability benefits and social care pathways**
- **Opportunities for community belonging and advocacy**

Without a proper assessment, these vital supports often remain out of reach. Misdiagnosis—or complete missed diagnosis—can have serious consequences. Furthermore, misdiagnosis or missed diagnosis can lead to inappropriate treatment approaches, particularly for co-occurring mental health conditions. For example, the therapeutic approaches that might be helpful for a neurotypical person experiencing anxiety may require significant adaptation for someone with autism. Understanding the autistic neurotype allows for more tailored and effective interventions across all domains of healthcare.

The UK perspective on autism assessment has several distinctive features that differentiate it from other international approaches.

- **ICD-11 vs. DSM-5-TR**: Unlike some international contexts that rely on the DSM-5-TR, UK clinicians primarily use the ICD-11. This influences diagnostic terminology and criteria, and it's essential to understand these nuances when assessing adults.
- **NHS Service Structure**: Most UK regions have specialist adult autism assessment teams, though **access varies geographically**, with significant differences in waiting times and service models. Navigating these systems is part of the clinical challenge.
- **NICE Guidelines**: NICE Clinical Guideline 142, updated in 2021, provides a UK-specific, evidence-based framework for autism diagnosis. It emphasizes **multi-disciplinary evaluation**, **comprehensive developmental history**, and consideration of co-occurring conditions.

Throughout this training, we will explore the practical application of these guidelines in clinical settings, the challenges of implementing best practices within resource constraints, and the evolving understanding of autism across the lifespan. We will pay particular attention to aspects of assessment that may be challenging for clinicians new to this field, including **recognizing autism in those who have developed sophisticated compensatory strategies**, **understanding**

the female phenotype, **distinguishing autism from other conditions with overlapping features**, and **conducting assessments with cultural sensitivity**.

By the conclusion of this training, you should feel equipped to approach adult autism assessment with greater confidence, clinical skill, and understanding of the unique needs of this population. You will understand the core components of a comprehensive assessment, the standardized tools available and their limitations, the process of clinical decision-making in complex cases, and the post-diagnostic support needs of adults receiving a diagnosis. Most importantly, you will appreciate the profound impact that skilled, sensitive assessment can have on the lives of adults who have spent years or decades without understanding any fundamental aspect of their neurological makeup.

CHAPTER 2

Overview of Autism Spectrum Disorder

Autism Spectrum Disorder (ASD) represents a complex neurodevelopmental condition characterized by persistent patterns of difference in two core domains: **social communication and interaction**, and **restricted, repetitive patterns of behaviour, interests, or activities**. To thoroughly understand ASD, we must appreciate it as a **lifelong neurobiological condition with early developmental origins** that manifests across multiple domains of functioning.

In the domain of social communication and interaction, individuals with ASD typically demonstrate qualitative differences rather than simple delays. These differences affect verbal and non-verbal communication and can manifest in various ways:

- Difficulty with the **reciprocal nature** of conversation.
- Challenges with **pragmatic language** (the social use of language).
- Limited or atypical use of **eye contact, facial expressions**, and **gestures**.
- Difficulty with the intuitive understanding of **social rules** and contexts.

These social communication differences exist on a spectrum—some individuals may appear aloof or uninterested in social interaction, while others may be highly socially motivated but struggle with the execution of social skills or understanding the unwritten rules of social engagement.

The second core domain involves restricted, repetitive patterns of behaviour, interests, or activities. This broad category encompasses several distinct manifestations: repetitive physical movements (sometimes called "stimming");

- Insistence on sameness and difficulty with transitions or changes in routine;
- Highly focused interests that are unusual in intensity or focus.
- Sensory processing differences, which may include hypersensitivity or hyposensitivity to sensory input across any sensory modality.

These features may serve various functions, including **self-regulation**, **anxiety management**, or simply reflecting **natural cognitive preferences for predictability and depth of focus.**

The prevalence of ASD in the UK adult population is estimated at approximately 1-2%, translating to over 700,000 adults in the UK. However, this figure may underestimate the true prevalence, as many adults remain undiagnosed, particularly those without intellectual disabilities and those who have developed effective compensatory strategies. Recent epidemiological research suggests the prevalence may be higher than previously thought, with some studies indicating rates approaching 2.5% in adult populations.

Historically, autism was diagnosed significantly more frequently in males than females, with ratios reported as high as 4:1 or even higher. However, contemporary research strongly suggests that this discrepancy reflects a systematic diagnostic bias rather than a true difference in prevalence. Females with autism often present differently from the traditionally recognized male phenotype on which early diagnostic criteria were based. Features commonly seen in autistic women and girls include:

- **Social camouflaging** and mimicry of neurotypical behaviors.
- **Subtler special interests**, often socially acceptable or age-appropriate in appearance.
- **Less overt repetitive behaviors**, which may be internalized or masked.

This "**female phenotype**" has been systematically under-recognized in diagnostic systems and clinical practice, leading to significant under-diagnosis in women and girls. Current research suggests that the true male-to-female ratio may be closer to 3:2 or even 1:1 when accounting for these diagnostic biases. As clinicians, developing a sophisticated understanding of how autism presents across genders is essential for accurate assessment.

The impact of ASD on adult life varies tremendously based on the individual's profile of strengths and challenges, cognitive abilities, presence of co-occurring conditions, environmental demands, and access to appropriate supports. In educational settings, adults with ASD may struggle with the social and sensory aspects of learning environments, group work, and implicit expectations, despite often having areas of significant academic strength. Employment statistics reveal concerning patterns, with only 21.7% of autistic adults in the UK in full-time employment—the lowest employment rate among all disability groups. This unemployment and underemployment often reflect social communication challenges in interviewing and workplace interactions, sensory barriers in work environments, and employers' lack of understanding rather than a lack of skills or qualifications.

In the domain of relationships, many autistic adults desire meaningful social and romantic connections but may struggle with the unwritten rules of relationship development and maintenance. Some may experience profound social isolation, while others may have relationships that are characterized by misunderstandings and difficulty with perspective-taking. **Independent living** can present challenges related to executive functioning difficulties, sensory sensitivities that affect daily activities like shopping or using public transportation, and the complex social navigation required for many aspects of adult life.

Autism Spectrum Disorder (ASD) is rarely a standalone diagnosis. It is frequently accompanied by co-occurring conditions that can significantly impact functioning and quality of life. These include **anxiety disorders** (occurring in up to 70% of autistic adults), **depression** (affecting approximately 40%), **ADHD** (co-occurring in 30-50%), and **specific learning difficulties including dyslexia or dyspraxia, may further impact daily functioning**. Physical health conditions are also more common, including **epilepsy, gastrointestinal problems**, **sleep disorders**, and **immune system differences**. The interaction between autism and these co-occurring conditions creates complex clinical presentations that require sophisticated assessment and understanding.

It is essential to recognize that autism exists as a spectrum not simply of "severity" but of diverse presentations. Each autistic individual has a unique profile of strengths and challenges that cannot be reduced to a linear concept of "mild" to "severe" autism. Some individuals may exhibit exceptional cognitive abilities in specific domains alongside significant challenges in others. Others may have more consistent profiles across domains but with specific areas of difficulty. Understanding this dimensional nature of autism is crucial for meaningful assessment and support planning.

Finally, perspectives on autism have evolved significantly in recent decades, with growing recognition of the neurodiversity paradigm, which conceptualizes autism as a natural variation in human neurocognitive functioning rather than inherently a disorder or deficit. This perspective acknowledges the genuine challenges associated with autism in neurotypically-designed environments while also recognizing the potential strengths and valuable cognitive differences that can accompany autism. As clinicians, balancing an understanding of the very real difficulties that bring adults to diagnostic services with respect for neurocognitive diversity is an important ethical consideration in assessment.

CHAPTER 3

The UK Assessment Framework

The assessment of autism spectrum disorder in adults in the United Kingdom follows a structured framework guided by national standards and pathways. As psychiatrists and trainees, understanding this framework is essential for delivering consistent, high-quality assessments that meet both clinical and service standards. The cornerstone of this framework is the **National Institute for Health and Care Excellence (NICE) Guideline NG142**: "*Autism Spectrum Disorder in adults: diagnosis and management*," which provides evidence-based recommendations for the identification, assessment, and diagnosis of autism in adults.

NICE Guideline NG142, last updated in 2021, outlines several key principles for autism assessment. The guidelines emphasize that assessment should be comprehensive, drawing on multiple sources of information including clinical interviews, observational assessment, and where possible, developmental history from informants who knew the person during childhood. The guidelines specifically recommend that autism-specific standardized instruments should be considered to support the assessment process, though they should not be relied upon alone for diagnosis. NICE also highlights the importance of a multidisciplinary approach, suggesting that assessment teams should include professionals with expertise in autism assessment across multiple domains of functioning.

The practical implementation of these guidelines occurs within the NHS pathway for adult autism assessment. This pathway typically begins with a **referral**, which may come from primary care (GP), secondary mental health services, learning disability services, or in some regions, through self-referral. Following referral, many services implement a **screening or triage process** to ensure that a full diagnostic assessment is appropriate. This may involve screening questionnaires such as the Autism Spectrum Quotient (AQ) or an initial appointment to clarify the presenting concerns and determine whether they align with potential autism spectrum features.

The structure of diagnostic services varies across the UK, creating a somewhat heterogeneous landscape of care. In some regions, individuals have access to specialized autism assessment centres that provide dedicated diagnostic services with teams of clinicians who focus exclusively on autism assessment. These specialist centres often have the advantage of concentrated expertise but may have longer waiting lists due to high demand. In other areas, assessment may be conducted within broader mental health services or neurodevelopmental teams, which may have less specialized autism expertise but potentially shorter waiting times. This regional variation means that the specific pathway a patient follows may differ depending on their geographic location, creating potential inequities in access and quality of assessment.

Regardless of the service structure, the multi-disciplinary team (MDT) model is widely regarded as best practice across the UK. The core disciplines typically involved include **psychiatry**, **clinical psychology**, **speech and language therapy (SLT)**, and **occupational therapy (OT)**, each bringing a distinct and valuable perspective to the assessment process. Psychiatrists play a particularly crucial role in several aspects of the assessment:

1. **Differential diagnosis**: Psychiatrists' broad training in various mental health conditions positions them to consider the full range of potential differential diagnoses and to recognize patterns of comorbidity. This expertise is essential in distinguishing autism from conditions with overlapping features and in recognizing when multiple conditions may be co-occurring.
2. **Medical assessment**: Psychiatrists can assess for potential medical conditions that may be relevant, either as part of a differential diagnosis or as co-occurring conditions that may impact functioning.
3. **Medication review and recommendations**: For patients already taking medications or those who may benefit from pharmacological approaches to co-occurring conditions, psychiatrists provide essential expertise in medication management.
4. **Integration of the biopsychosocial model**: Psychiatrists' training in the biopsychosocial model enables them to consider the interaction between biological factors, psychological processes, and social context in understanding a person's presentation.
5. **Leading the diagnostic decision-making process**: In many teams, consultant psychiatrists hold ultimate clinical responsibility for diagnostic decisions, synthesizing information from multiple sources and team members to reach a diagnostic conclusion.

The typical referral pathways into autism assessment services vary across the UK but generally include:

1. **Primary care referrals**: General practitioners may refer patients who present with features suggestive of autism or who specifically request an autism assessment. The quality of these referrals can vary significantly based on the GP's knowledge of autism, highlighting the importance of clear referral criteria and education for primary care providers.
2. **Secondary mental health service referrals**: Many adults with undiagnosed autism initially present to mental health services with anxiety, depression, or other mental health conditions. Clinicians in these services may recognize autism features underlying these presentations and refer for specialized assessment.
3. **Self-referral:** Some regions have implemented self-referral pathways, allowing individuals to directly access autism assessment services without requiring a professional referral. This approach can reduce barriers to diagnosis but requires robust triage processes to manage service demand.
4. **Educational institution or employer referrals:** In some cases, universities, colleges, or employers may suggest assessment, though these would typically be channelled through primary care.
5. **Learning disability services:** For adults with intellectual disabilities, referrals often come through learning disability teams who identify features consistent with autism.

While the **NICE guidelines (NG142)** and **NHS pathways** provide a structured and evidence-based framework for adult autism assessment, their practical implementation across the UK faces several persistent challenges. Perhaps the most significant is the **lengthy waiting times for assessment**, which in some regions exceed two years from referral to assessment. These delays reflect both high demand for diagnostic services and limited resources, creating significant barriers to timely diagnosis. Additionally, the **transition between child and adult services** remains problematic, with many young people facing disruption in their care pathway as they move between service structures at age 18.

Another significant challenge is ensuring **cultural sensitivity and accessibility in assessment processes**. The UK's diverse population requires assessment approaches that can distinguish between cultural differences and autism features, and that are accessible to individuals from various linguistic and cultural backgrounds. Current standardized instruments have limited cross-cultural validation, creating potential for bias in assessment.

Despite these challenges, the UK framework for autism assessment provides a structured approach that, when implemented effectively, enables comprehensive, evidence-based assessment. As clinicians working within this framework, understanding both its strengths and limitations is essential for providing high-quality assessments that serve the needs of adults seeking autism diagnosis.

CHAPTER 4

Pre-Assessment Considerations

Before initiating a comprehensive autism assessment with an adult, several critical pre-assessment considerations must be addressed to ensure the process is clinically appropriate, ethically sound, and optimally informative. These preparatory steps lay the foundation for a successful assessment and help establish the conditions under which accurate diagnostic conclusions can be reached.

The first gate of the diagnostic pathway is referral screening, which serves as an initial filter to determine whether a full autism assessment is warranted. Given the significant resource investment of a comprehensive assessment and the lengthy waiting lists in many UK services, effective screening is essential for appropriate **prioritisation and allocation** of limited clinical capacity.. Referral screening typically involves reviewing the referral information against service criteria and may include preliminary screening measures such as the Autism Spectrum Quotient (AQ) or other structured questionnaires. When evaluating referrals, clinicians should look for descriptions of difficulties in social communication and interaction alongside restricted, repetitive patterns of behaviour or interests. However, it's important to recognize that referrers may not use autism-specific terminology, and features may be described in various ways that nonetheless suggest autism spectrum characteristics(e.g., "struggles with socialising," "rigid routines," or "feels different from others"). Skilled clinicians must learn to **interpret these descriptions through a neurodevelopmental lens**, identifying potential indicators of autism even when the language is non-specialist.

Importantly, screening should be approached with awareness of potential biases that might lead to missed cases. For example, well-educated adults with strong verbal abilities may not initially appear to meet criteria despite having significant social and sensory challenges. Similarly, women or gender-diverse individuals with autism often present differently from the traditional male phenotype against which many screening tools were developed. Their challenges may be subtler, more internalized, or more socially camouflaged. Effective screening balances the need for appropriate service utilization with sensitivity to the diverse presentations of autism across different demographic groups.

Once a referral is accepted for assessment, comprehensive information gathering becomes essential. This process should begin well before the first face-to-face assessment session. Requesting and reviewing records from education, previous healthcare contacts, and where applicable, employment support services provide valuable historical context and may reveal patterns consistent with autism that have been present but not previously recognized as such. School reports are particularly valuable, as they often contain observations about social interaction, responses to changes in routine, and special interests that may support an autism diagnosis, even when autism was not considered at the time.

For younger adults (typically aged 17-25), educational records are often more readily available and may contain more detailed information about developmental patterns. For older adults, educational records may be more difficult to obtain, making other sources of historical information, such as employment records, previous psychiatric assessments, or family accounts, more important. When gathering such information, it's essential to obtain appropriate consent and to explain clearly how this information will be used in the assessment process. Transparency fosters trust and helps set expectations around the collaborative nature of the diagnostic process.

Consent and capacity considerations are paramount in adult autism assessment. While most adults referred for autism assessment will have capacity to consent to the process, this should never be assumed without consideration. Some adults with autism may also have intellectual disabilities or mental health conditions that affect their capacity to make specific decisions about assessment. In such cases, the principles of the **Mental Capacity Act 2005** must be followed, ensuring that:

1. Capacity is presumed unless there is evidence to the contrary
2. All practicable steps are taken to support the person to make their own decision
3. People have the right to make unwise decisions if they have capacity
4. Any decision made on behalf of someone lacking capacity must be in their best interests
5. Any intervention should be the least restrictive of their rights and freedoms

In practical terms, ensuring informed consent means providing clear, accessible information about what the assessment will involve, how information will be used, the potential outcomes (including both the benefits and potential challenges of receiving an autism diagnosis), and any limits to confidentiality. This information should be provided in formats appropriate to the individual's communication preferences and processing style, which might include written information, visual supports, or recorded explanations that can be reviewed multiple times.

Identifying support needs for the assessment process itself is another crucial pre-assessment consideration. Adults with possible autism may find aspects of the assessment process challenging due to sensory sensitivities, anxiety in unfamiliar social situations, difficulty with open-ended questions, or executive functioning challenges that affect planning and organization. Proactively identifying and addressing these potential barriers can significantly improve the quality and validity of the assessment. Practical accommodations might include:

- Providing detailed information about what to expect during the assessment, including the physical environment, the people who will be present, and the types of activities involved
- Offering choices about the timing and pacing of assessment sessions (e.g., shorter, more frequent sessions versus longer, fewer sessions)
- Adapting the physical environment to minimize sensory discomfort (e.g., reducing fluorescent lighting, minimizing background noise, allowing for movement breaks)
- Using visual supports or written questions to supplement verbal interaction
- Allowing the person to bring a trusted support person if desired
- Being flexible about the mode of assessment (e.g., considering remote options for portions of the assessment if in-person interaction is particularly challenging)

Cultural considerations represent a particularly important aspect of pre-assessment planning. Autism presents across all cultural, ethnic, and socioeconomic groups, but its recognition and interpretation may be significantly influenced by cultural factors. Behaviours that might be interpreted as autism features in one cultural context might be understood differently in another. For example, norms regarding eye contact, conversational style, emotional expression, and relationship to authority figures vary substantially across cultures. Additionally, the concept of neurodevelopmental difference itself is understood and stigmatized differently across cultural contexts, affecting how individuals and families may approach the assessment process.

To address these cultural dimensions, pre-assessment planning should include:

1. Gathering information about the person's cultural background and understanding how this might influence the presentation and interpretation of behaviours

2. Considering whether standardized assessment instruments have been validated in the cultural context relevant to the individual
3. Ensuring access to appropriate interpretation services if there are language differences, recognizing that autism assessment requires nuanced understanding of communication that goes beyond simple translation
4. Being aware of how cultural factors might influence the person's and their family's understanding of and attitudes toward autism diagnosis
5. Adapting the explanation of the assessment process and potential outcomes to align with cultural understandings while still providing accurate clinical information

Finally, practical logistics must be addressed before beginning the assessment. This includes scheduling considerations, arrangement of appropriate space and materials, coordination among team members if a multi-disciplinary approach is being used, and ensuring that any required standardized assessment materials are available and in languages appropriate to the person being assessed. While seemingly mundane, these practical considerations can significantly impact the quality of the assessment and the experience of the person being assessed.

Thorough attention to these pre-assessment considerations not only improves the technical quality of the assessment but also demonstrates respect for the individual's autonomy, preferences, and unique context. This person-centred approach aligns with both ethical practice and the NICE quality standard that emphasizes the importance of individualized, accessible assessment processes.

CHAPTER 5

ASD Assessment Timeline

A comprehensive autism spectrum disorder (ASD) assessment for adults follows a structured timeline that typically spans multiple sessions and stages. Understanding this timeline is essential for effective service planning, managing patient expectations, and ensuring thorough assessment without unnecessary delays. While there is some variation in assessment timelines across different services within the UK, the following represents a standard model aligned with NICE guidelines and best clinical practices.

The assessment process usually begins with **initial screening**, which typically encompasses one to two sessions. This preliminary phase serves several important functions. First, it allows clinicians to **determine whether a full autism assessment is warranted** based on the presenting concerns and symptoms. During these initial sessions, clinicians **gather basic demographic information and conduct a preliminary exploration** of the individual's current difficulties and developmental history. **Screening tools such as the Autism Spectrum Quotient (AQ) may be administered**, though it's important to note that these are not diagnostic in isolation. These initial sessions also provide an opportunity to **establish rapport** with the individual, explain the assessment process in detail, and address any questions or concerns they may have about the diagnostic journey.

In some services, particularly those with significant waiting lists, this screening phase may be separated from the full assessment by a substantial waiting period. During this waiting time, individuals may be directed to psychoeducational resources about autism or to support groups for those awaiting diagnosis. Some services also use this period to request additional information, such as educational records or developmental histories from family members, which can inform the subsequent comprehensive assessment.

The comprehensive assessment itself typically encompasses three to five sessions, though this can vary based on the individual's presentation, the assessment approach used, and service-specific protocols. These sessions are usually spaced over several weeks, allowing time for information processing, reflection, and the gathering of additional information between appointments. The spacing of appointments also provides opportunities to observe the individual in different states (e.g., varying energy or anxiety levels) and to assess the consistency of autism features across different contexts and times.

The comprehensive assessment sessions typically include:

1. **Detailed developmental history interview**: This session focuses on early development, including language acquisition, social development, play patterns, sensory sensitivities, and the emergence of restricted or repetitive behaviours. When possible, this history is gathered from both the individual and informants who knew them during childhood.
2. **Current functioning assessment**: This session explores current patterns of social communication, relationships, daily living skills, sensory sensitivities, special interests, and routines. This assessment typically includes both structured interview components and more naturalistic observation of social communication during the session itself.
3. **Administration of standardized instruments**: Depending on the service protocol, one or more sessions may be dedicated to administering standardized assessment tools such as the Autism Diagnostic Observation Schedule, Second Edition (ADOS-2) or other structured assessment measures.
4. **Cognitive assessment**: When indicated, a cognitive assessment may be included to understand the individual's intellectual profile, which can inform interpretation of social communication patterns and support planning.
5. **Functional impact assessment**: This component explores how the potential autism features impact the individual's daily functioning across domains such as education, employment, independent living, and relationships.

Parallel to these direct assessment sessions, the collection of collateral information occurs. This includes gathering information from multiple sources to develop a comprehensive understanding of the individual across different contexts and developmental periods. Sources of collateral information may include:

- Written reports from schools, universities, or workplaces
- Medical records from previous healthcare providers
- Questionnaires completed by family members, partners, or close friends
- Direct interviews with informants (in person, by phone, or via video conference)

- Observations in naturalistic settings (though this is less common in adult assessment)

Collateral Information and Diagnostic Formulation in Adult Autism Assessment

The collection of collateral development information is particularly important in adult assessment, as retrospective recall of developmental history may be challenging, and individuals with possible autism may have limited insight into some of their social communication patterns. However, gathering collateral information for adults can be challenging when parents are no longer living or contactable, or when individuals have limited contact with family members who knew them during childhood. In such cases, creative approaches to gathering historical information become necessary, such as reviewing old school reports, photographs, home videos, or speaking with extended family members or long-term friends.

Following the completion of all assessment components including clinical interviews, observational tools, screening measures, and review of historical information, the process moves to the **formulation and diagnostic decision-making phase**. In multidisciplinary services, these discussions bring together observations and information gathered by different team members to develop an integrated understanding of the individual's presentation. The formulation process considers how the various features observed align with diagnostic criteria for autism, explores alternative explanations for the presenting difficulties, and addresses questions of comorbidity. These team discussions typically last 1-2 hours and are a critical component of the diagnostic decision-making process.

After reaching diagnostic conclusions, a feedback session is arranged with the individual. This crucial session, typically lasting 60-90 minutes, involves sharing the findings of the assessment in a clear, sensitive manner. The feedback session should:

- Review the assessment process that was undertaken
- Explain the diagnostic conclusion and the evidence supporting it
- Discuss the implications of the diagnosis (or alternative conclusions if autism is not diagnosed)
- Provide opportunity for questions and emotional processing
- Outline recommendations and next steps
- Provide relevant resources and information

This feedback session is not merely an information-giving exercise but a therapeutic interaction that requires careful preparation and skill. The manner in which diagnostic information is shared can significantly impact how the individual processes and integrates this information into their self-understanding. Many adults report that the feedback session is one of the most significant aspects of the entire assessment process.

Following the feedback session, report writing takes place. The diagnostic report serves as a formal record of the assessment findings and recommendations. In accordance with NICE guidelines, this report should be completed promptly following the feedback session, ideally within 4-6 weeks. The report should be shared with the individual and, with their consent, relevant healthcare providers and support services. The report serves multiple purposes: **documenting the diagnostic decision, providing a reference for the individual to understand their diagnosis, supporting applications for accommodations or benefits**, and **informing future healthcare providers about the individual's needs.**

The final phase of the assessment timeline involves post-diagnostic support. While this extends beyond the assessment itself, planning for post-diagnostic support should be integrated into the assessment process. Depending on local service configurations, this may include:

- Referral to post-diagnostic groups or courses
- Connection with autism-specific support services
- Workplace or educational accommodation recommendations
- Referrals for specific interventions for co-occurring conditions
- Benefits or funding support applications
- Follow-up appointments to address questions that arise after diagnosis

The entire assessment timeline, from initial screening to completion of the report, typically spans 3-6 months in well-resourced services, though in many NHS services, waiting lists for initial assessment can extend this timeline significantly. Throughout this process, clear communication about timeframes and next steps is essential for maintaining engagement and managing expectations.

This structured timeline ensures that assessment is comprehensive, incorporates multiple sources of information, and leads to well-supported diagnostic conclusions. While resource constraints may create pressure to abbreviate this process, maintaining the integrity of the full assessment timeline is important for diagnostic accuracy and for providing individuals with a thorough understanding of their neurological profile.

CHAPTER 6

The Multi-Dimensional Assessment Approach

Autism Spectrum Disorder (ASD) is a complex, multifaceted condition that affects individuals across numerous domains of functioning. To effectively assess for ASD in adults, a multi-dimensional approach is essential—one that captures the diverse manifestations of autism across different contexts, throughout development, and in relation to the individual's overall neuropsychological profile. This comprehensive approach ensures that diagnostic decisions are based on a rich, contextual understanding rather than isolated observations or self-reports.

The cornerstone of any autism assessment is the clinical interview, which provides both current and historical information essential for diagnostic decision-making. A well-conducted clinical interview explores the individual's developmental history, focusing on early indicators of social communication differences and restricted or repetitive patterns of behaviour. For adults, this historical information can be challenging to obtain, particularly for older adults whose parents may no longer be available for interview. In such cases, creative approaches may be needed, such as reviewing school reports, examining childhood photographs or videos, or speaking with siblings or other relatives who knew the person during childhood.

The clinical interview also examines current functioning across multiple domains, including social relationships, communication patterns, sensory sensitivities, special interests, and daily living skills. Throughout the interview, the clinician should be attentive not only to the content of responses but also to qualitative aspects of communication that may reflect autism features, such as unusual prosody, limited facial expression, difficulty with narrative coherence, or literal interpretation of questions. The manner in which information is conveyed often provides as much diagnostic information as the content itself.

While the clinical interview provides rich qualitative data, standardized instruments offer structured, empirically validated approaches to assessment.

These instruments fall into several categories, each contributing distinct information to the diagnostic process:

The **Autism Diagnostic Observation Schedule, Second Edition (ADOS-2)** is considered the gold standard observational assessment for autism. This semi-structured, standardized protocol creates social presses that allow the examiner to observe how the individual navigates various social situations. For adults, Module 4 is typically used, which includes activities such as conversation, description of a picture, telling a story from a book, discussing emotions, demonstrating a task, and discussing social challenges. Throughout these activities, the examiner rates the individual's social communication, reciprocal interaction, imagination, and stereotyped behaviours or restricted interests. The structured nature of the ADOS-2 allows for comparison to normative data and provides standardized criteria for interpreting observations.

It is essential to emphasize that proper training and certification are required to administer and interpret the ADOS-2. This typically involves attending a clinical training workshop, completing practice administrations, and achieving reliability with established scoring standards. Without this formal training, the validity of ADOS-2 results is compromised, and its use would not meet the standards outlined in NICE guidelines.

The **Autism Diagnostic Interview-Revised (ADI-R)** provides a complementary assessment approach, focusing on developmental history as reported by parents or other long-term caregivers. This comprehensive interview explores early development and behaviour in the domains of social interaction, communication, and restricted or repetitive behaviours. The ADI-R's structured format ensures systematic coverage of key developmental indicators of autism and provides algorithms for evaluating the pattern of responses against diagnostic criteria. Like the ADOS-2, the ADI-R requires formal training and certification for valid administration and interpretation.

While the ADI-R was developed primarily for childhood assessment, it can be adapted for adult assessment when informants with knowledge of the person's early development are available. However, the retrospective nature of this information introduces potential recall biases, particularly when asking parents to remember details from several decades earlier. Despite these limitations, the developmental perspective provided by the ADI-R offers crucial information that cannot be obtained through current observation alone.

In addition to these autism-specific instruments, various questionnaires provide valuable self-report and informant-report data. These include measures such as:

- **The Autism Spectrum Quotient (AQ)**, which assesses autistic traits across social skills, attention switching, attention to detail, communication, and imagination.
- **The Ritvo Autism Asperger Diagnostic Scale-Revised (RAADS-R)**, which examines social relatedness, circumscribed interests, language, and sensory-motor features.
- **The Social Responsiveness Scale-2 (SRS-2)**, which measures social awareness, social cognition, social communication, social motivation, and restricted interests/repetitive behaviours.

These questionnaires can be completed by the individual being assessed and by informants who know them well, providing multiple perspectives on autism-related behaviours. However, it is crucial to recognize that these instruments were developed primarily with male samples and may not be equally sensitive to female presentations of autism. Furthermore, individuals with autism may have limited insight into some of their social communication patterns, potentially affecting the validity of self-report measures. Despite these limitations, questionnaires provide a time-efficient method for gathering structured information that can inform the broader assessment process.

Observational assessment extends beyond standardized measures like the ADOS-2 to include both structured and naturalistic observation. Structured observation involves creating specific social situations or tasks that elicit behaviours relevant to diagnosis, such as unstructured conversation, problem-solving tasks, or group interactions. Naturalistic observation, while more challenging in adult assessment, might include observing the individual in waiting rooms, during transitions between assessment components, or in community settings when possible. Both approaches provide opportunities to observe spontaneous behaviour that may not be captured in formal testing situations.

When appropriate, **cognitive assessment** can provide valuable information about the individual's intellectual profile, which may influence the presentation of autism features and inform support planning. Cognitive assessment typically includes measures of verbal and non-verbal intelligence, working memory, processing speed, and executive functioning. Distinctive cognitive profiles are often associated with autism, such as discrepancies between verbal and perceptual abilities, strengths in specific domains like visuospatial processing or rote memory, and challenges in areas requiring cognitive flexibility or social cognition. Understanding these cognitive patterns helps contextualize social communication differences and can identify specific strengths that may be leveraged in intervention planning.

Functional assessment examines how potential autism features impact daily living across domains such as education, employment, independent living, and relationships. This assessment may include structured measures of adaptive functioning, such as the **Adaptive Behaviour Assessment System** or the **Vineland Adaptive Behaviour Scales**, as well as detailed discussion of real-world challenges and accommodations. Functional assessment is particularly important in adult assessment, as it highlights the practical implications of autism features and informs recommendations for support. NICE guidelines emphasize the importance of assessing functional impact, noting that diagnosis should consider not only the presence of autism features but also their effect on the individual's life.

In some cases, medical examination may be indicated as part of the assessment process. This might include genetic testing, particularly when there are dysmorphic features, a family history of genetic conditions, or intellectual disability of unknown ethology. Neurological examination may be warranted when there are concerns about seizures, motor coordination problems, or other neurological symptoms. Sensory assessments, conducted by occupational therapists, can provide detailed information about sensory processing patterns that may impact daily functioning. These medical components are not routine in all adult autism assessments but should be considered based on the individual's presentation and history.

The integration of information from these multiple assessment dimensions requires clinical judgment and team discussion. No single assessment component is sufficient for diagnosis, and discrepancies between different sources of information are common. For example, an individual may score above threshold on self-report measures but below threshold on observational assessment, or vice versa. Such discrepancies do not invalidate the assessment but rather highlight the complex, context-dependent nature of autism features and the importance of comprehensive assessment across multiple domains.

The multi-dimensional approach described here aligns with NICE guidelines, which emphasize that diagnosis should not rely on any single autism-specific instrument but should integrate information from multiple sources. This comprehensive approach ensures that diagnostic decisions are based on a thorough understanding of the individual's developmental history, current functioning, and the impact of autism features on their life. It also recognizes the heterogeneity of autism presentations and the need for individualized assessment approaches that capture each person's unique profile of strengths and challenges.

CHAPTER 7
Essential Clinical Interview Components

The clinical interview forms the cornerstone of autism assessment in adults, providing crucial information about developmental history, current functioning, and the subjective experience of autism features. While standardized instruments offer structured evaluation, the clinical interview allows for a nuanced exploration of the individual's unique presentation and life context. A well-conducted clinical interview not only gathers essential diagnostic information but also establishes rapport, validates the individual's experiences, and lays the foundation for post-diagnostic support planning. The following components are essential to include in the clinical interview portion of an autism assessment.

The developmental history component of the interview aims to identify early indicators of autism that may have been present from childhood. This retrospective exploration is crucial for establishing the developmental nature of autism, which is a defining characteristic of the condition. Key aspects of development to explore include early developmental milestones, particularly in the domains of motor skills, language acquisition, and social development. While gross delays in these areas are not universal in autism, subtle differences in the quality or pattern of development may be informative. For example, an individual may have acquired language at a typical age but shown unusual patterns such as formal or pedantic speech, pronoun reversals, or difficulties with the pragmatic aspects of language despite strong vocabulary.

The interview should explore early social development in detail, including how the individual interacted with peers and adults, whether they sought shared experiences, how they engaged in play, and whether they formed age-appropriate friendships. Particular attention should be paid to imitation, joint attention, social reciprocity, and understanding of social rules, as differences in these areas may indicate early social communication challenges consistent with autism. It's important to recognize that some individuals with autism, particularly those without intellectual disabilities, may have developed compensatory strategies that masked their social difficulties during structured school activities but became more apparent during unstructured social time or as social demands increased with age.

Educational history provides valuable information about academic strengths and challenges, social experiences in school, responses to transitions, and any support or accommodations received. The interview should explore patterns across different educational stages and settings, noting any consistent difficulties or environments in which the individual particularly thrived or struggled. School reports can provide contemporaneous observations of behaviours that may reflect autism features, even if autism was not considered at the time. For example, comments about being "in their own world," having difficulty working in groups, becoming upset with changes in routine, or showing intense focus on particular topics may suggest unrecognized autism features.

The relationship history component explores the individual's experiences with friendships, romantic relationships, and family dynamics. This includes examining the quantity and quality of relationships, patterns of relationship development and maintenance, and understanding of social dynamics. Many adults with undiagnosed autism report a history of relationship difficulties, including misunderstandings, feeling "different" from peers, difficulty reading social cues, or struggling to maintain relationships despite genuine interest in social connection. Others may describe limited interest in social relationships or preference for solitary activities. Both patterns can be consistent with autism, reflecting different manifestations of social communication differences.

The family history exploration should include questions about neurodevelopmental and mental health conditions in biological relatives, as autism has a strong genetic component. A family history of diagnosed or suspected autism, attention deficit hyperactivity disorder, specific learning difficulties, or language disorders may increase the likelihood of autism in the individual being assessed. Additionally, exploring the family environment and relationship patterns can provide context for understanding how autism features may have been supported, accommodated, or perhaps masked within the family system.

The medical history review should encompass relevant physical and mental health conditions, medications, and previous healthcare contacts. Certain medical conditions occur more frequently in autism, including epilepsy, gastrointestinal disorders, sleep disturbances, and immune system differences. A history of multiple mental health diagnoses or treatments with limited response might suggest that underlying autism has been overlooked. Additionally, sensory sensitivities or motor coordination difficulties may have led to medical consultations without the connection to potential autism being recognized.

The exploration of current functioning should cover multiple domains of daily life, including:

1. **Social communication and relationships**: Current social network, communication style, understanding of social rules and norms, perspective-taking abilities, and any difficulties in social contexts.
2. **Education or employment**: Current activities, strengths and challenges in these settings, accommodations needed, and relationships with colleagues or fellow students.
3. **Independent living skills**: Ability to manage daily responsibilities, executive functioning in everyday tasks, organization of living space, and any support needed.
4. **Special interests and routines**: Current interests in terms of content, intensity, and social sharing; daily routines and response to changes or interruptions; and repetitive behaviours or sensory seeking activities.
5. **Sensory experiences**: Sensitivities or seeking behaviours across sensory domains (auditory, visual, tactile, olfactory, gustatory, proprioceptive, vestibular) and their impact on daily functioning.
6. **Emotional regulation**: Recognition and management of emotions, responses to stress, and coping strategies.

Throughout the interview, attention should be paid not only to the content of responses but also to qualitative aspects of communication that may reflect autism features, such as:

- Eye contact patterns and quality
- Facial expressiveness and coordination with verbal content
- Prosody, volume, and rhythm of speech
- Use of gesture and body language
- Narrative coherence and relevance
- Turn-taking in conversation
- Understanding of figurative language or humour
- Response to social cues from the interviewer

The presenting concerns component explores the individual's own understanding of their difficulties and reasons for seeking assessment. This provides insight into self-awareness and helps focus the assessment on areas of particular relevance to the individual. Some adults seeking autism assessment will have conducted extensive research and identify strongly with autism characteristics, while others may have limited understanding of autism but have been encouraged to seek assessment by healthcare professionals, family members, or employers. Understanding this context helps tailor the assessment approach and informs how findings will be shared.

When conducting the clinical interview, several methodological considerations are important:

1. **Structure and flexibility**: While covering all essential components, the interview should remain flexible enough to follow important lines of inquiry as they emerge and to adapt to the individual's communication style and needs.
2. **Concrete questioning**: Many individuals with autism benefit from specific, concrete questions rather than abstract or open-ended inquiries. For example, asking "Can you tell me about a specific situation where you found it difficult to understand what someone else was thinking?" may elicit more informative responses than "How is your social understanding?"
3. **Processing time**: Allowing adequate time for processing questions and formulating responses is essential, as many individuals with autism require more time to process social information and organize their thoughts, particularly around abstract or emotional topics.
4. **Visual supports**: Some individuals may benefit from visual timelines, rating scales, or written questions to support the interview process, reducing the social and language processing demands.
5. **Sensory considerations**: Attention to the interview environment, including lighting, background noise, seating arrangements, and break opportunities, can significantly affect the individual's comfort and ability to engage effectively.
6. **Recognition of masking**: Many adults with autism, particularly women and those with higher cognitive abilities, may have developed sophisticated strategies to mask their autism features in formal situations like an assessment. The interviewer should be attuned to subtle indicators of effort, fatigue, or inconsistencies between reported difficulties and observed presentation.

The clinical interview for adult autism assessment requires considerable skill, combining structured information gathering with sensitive atonement to the individual's experience and presentation. When conducted effectively, it provides a rich foundation of information that, combined with standardized assessments and collateral reports, enables accurate diagnostic formulation and meaningful support recommendations.

CHAPTER 8

Specialized Instruments - Introduction

Standardized assessment instruments play a crucial role in the comprehensive assessment of autism spectrum disorder in adults. These instruments provide structured, empirically validated approaches to gathering and interpreting information, complementing the clinical interview and observational data with quantifiable measures that can be compared to normative standards. When used appropriately, standardized instruments enhance the reliability and validity of the assessment process, reducing the potential for subjective bias and providing a common language for communicating findings across professionals and services.

The purpose of standardized assessment extends beyond simply confirming or ruling out a diagnosis. These instruments provide detailed information about the specific profile of autism features, highlighting areas of particular strength or challenge that can inform individualized support planning. They offer a systematic approach to gathering information across multiple domains, ensuring comprehensive coverage of diagnostic criteria. Additionally, standardized measures can help differentiate autism from conditions with overlapping features and identify patterns of comorbidity that might otherwise be overlooked.

However, clinicians must approach standardized instruments with a clear understanding of their limitations and potential biases. Most autism assessment tools were developed and validated primarily with male samples, often those with more obvious presentations of autism. This historical bias creates significant challenges when assessing women and individuals with more subtle presentations, as the instruments may lack sensitivity to these manifestations of autism. Recent research has highlighted substantial gender differences in autism presentation, with females often showing more sophisticated social camouflaging, different patterns of special interests, and less obvious repetitive behaviours. Standard instruments may fail to capture these gender-specific presentations, leading to potential underdiagnosis in females.

Cultural biases represent another significant limitation of standardized instruments. Most measures were developed in Western, predominantly white populations, with limited cross-cultural validation. Cultural differences in communication styles, social norms, eye contact, emotional expression, and relationship to authority figures can significantly influence responses to assessment items, potentially leading to misinterpretation of culturally normative behaviours as autism features—or conversely, missing autism features that present differently across cultural contexts. These cultural considerations are particularly important in the diverse UK population, where assessment must be culturally sensitive and appropriate.

Many standardized instruments were initially developed for childhood assessment and later adapted for adults. These adaptations may not fully capture the developmental changes in autism presentation across the lifespan or the sophisticated compensatory strategies that many adults develop. Items designed to detect autism features in children may lack sensitivity to the more subtle, adapted presentations common in adults, particularly those with higher cognitive abilities who have developed strategies to navigate social demands.

The interpretation of standardized assessment results requires clinical expertise and contextual understanding. Scores and classifications should never be applied mechanistically but must be interpreted in light of the individual's developmental history, current functioning, and specific assessment context. For example, an individual who scores below the clinical threshold on a standardized instrument may nonetheless meet diagnostic criteria based on developmental history and functional impact. Conversely, elevated scores on self-report measures may sometimes reflect conditions other than autism, such as social anxiety or schizotypal traits, highlighting the importance of comprehensive assessment rather than reliance on any single measure.

In the UK context, consideration of appropriate norms is essential when interpreting standardized measures. While some instruments have UK-specific normative data, many rely on norms developed in other countries, predominantly the United States. These international norms may not fully reflect the UK population, potentially affecting the accuracy of classification. When UK norms are available, they should be preferred, but clinicians should always maintain awareness of the normative context when interpreting results.

The selection of specific instruments should be guided by several criteria, tailored to the individual being assessed:

1. **Age appropriateness**: Instruments should be selected that are validated for the age range of the individual. For those in the transitional age range (late adolescence/early adulthood), careful consideration should be given to whether adult or adolescent measures are more appropriate based on developmental stage rather than chronological age alone.

2. **Verbal ability**: The individual's language skills should inform the choice of assessment measures. For adults with limited verbal abilities, instruments that do not rely heavily on expressive language should be selected. Conversely, for highly verbal individuals, measures sensitive to subtle pragmatic language differences are important.
3. **Purpose of assessment**: The specific questions driving the assessment should influence instrument selection. If educational accommodations are a primary concern, measures that provide detailed information about learning style and executive functioning may be prioritized. If the focus is on employment support, instruments examining social communication in workplace contexts might be more relevant.
4. **Available informants**: The selection of instruments should consider the availability of parents, partners, or other informants who can provide historical or current observational information. When informants are limited, greater emphasis may be placed on self-report and direct observational measures.
5. **Cultural and linguistic considerations**: Instruments should be selected that have been validated, when possible, in the cultural and linguistic context of the individual being assessed. When using instruments across cultural contexts, potential biases should be explicitly considered in interpretation.

Training requirements for standardized instruments vary, but many require formal certification to ensure reliable administration and scoring. The **ADOS-2** and **ADI-R**, in particular, require specific training and demonstration of competency before use in clinical practice. This training typically involves:

1. Attending a clinical training workshop delivered by certified trainers
2. Completing practice administrations under supervision
3. Demonstrating reliability in scoring compared to established standards
4. Maintaining skills through regular use and refresh training

These training requirements reflect the complexity of these instruments and the potential for administration or interpretation errors without proper preparation. Services offering autism assessment should ensure that clinicians using standardized instruments have completed all required training and maintain their skills through regular practice and supervision.

Access to Training and Practical Use of Standardized Instruments in the UK

In the UK, access to training for specialized instruments has historically been limited, with courses offered rarely and often at significant cost. This has created barriers to the widespread implementation of gold-standard assessment approaches, particularly in services with limited resources. Recent initiatives have aimed to increase training accessibility, including regional training hubs and distance learning options, but access remains a challenge in some areas. Services planning to implement comprehensive autism assessment should budget for both the initial training costs and ongoing maintenance of skills.

The implementation of standardized instruments must be balanced with practical constraints within clinical services. The time required for administration, scoring, and interpretation of comprehensive measures like the **ADOS-2** and **ADI-R** is substantial, typically requiring 2-3 hours each when including preparation and documentation. In resource-limited settings, strategic decisions may be needed about which instruments to prioritize, perhaps reserving the most time-intensive measures for complex or ambiguous cases while using briefer screening tools for more straightforward presentations.

Despite these limitations and practical challenges, standardized instruments remain an essential component of comprehensive autism assessment when used appropriately as part of a multi-method approach. They provide structure, empirical grounding, and systematic coverage of relevant domains that enhance the overall quality of assessment. The skilled integration of standardized measures with clinical interview, observational data, and developmental history allows for diagnostic decisions that reflect both empirical evidence and clinical expertise, ultimately serving the needs of adults seeking autism assessment.

CHAPTER 9

ADOS-2 (Autism Diagnostic Observation Schedule, 2nd Edition)

The **Autism Diagnostic Observation Schedule, Second Edition (ADOS-2)** represents the gold standard observational assessment instrument for autism spectrum disorder across the lifespan. Developed by Catherine Lord and her colleagues, the ADOS-2 provides a semi-structured, standardized context for observing social communication, interaction, play, and restricted and repetitive behaviours. For clinicians conducting adult autism assessments, a thorough understanding of this instrument—including its structure, administration, scoring, and interpretation—is essential for implementing evidence-based assessment practices.

The primary purpose of the ADOS-2 is to create a standardized context in which the clinician can directly observe behaviours relevant to autism diagnosis. While clinical interviews provide valuable information about reported behaviours, the ADOS-2 allows for direct observation of how the individual navigates social interactions in real time. This standardized observational approach offers several advantages:

- It creates consistent social presses across different individuals being assessed.
- It allows comparison to normative data; it reduces reliance on self-report or retrospective recall.
- It provides opportunities to observe subtle qualitative features of social communication that may not be captured in interviews.

It cannot be emphasized strongly enough that formal certification is absolutely mandatory for using the ADOS-2 in clinical practice. This is not simply a professional recommendation but an essential requirement for valid and reliable use of the instrument. The complexity of administration, scoring, and interpretation necessitates specialized training to ensure standardized implementation and accurate clinical conclusions. Formal ADOS-2 training typically involves:

1. A comprehensive clinical training workshop (typically 2-3 days) covering the theoretical background, administration procedures, and scoring conventions
2. Practice administrations with supervision and feedback
3. Demonstration of scoring reliability compared to established standards, often through coding of video-recorded administrations
4. Ongoing maintenance of skills through regular use and periodic refresher training

In the UK, ADOS-2 training is offered through several providers, including university-based research centres and private training organizations. The training represents a significant investment of time and resources, but it is essential for services offering autism assessment. Using the ADOS-2 without proper training compromises the validity of results and would not meet the standards outlined in NICE guidelines.

The ADOS-2 is structured into four modules, each designed for individuals at different developmental and language levels. For adult assessment, Module 4 is most commonly used, as it is designed for verbally fluent adolescents and adults. However, for adults with limited language or intellectual disabilities, Module 1 (preverbal/single words), Module 2 (phrase speech), or Module 3 (fluent speech - child/adolescent) may be more appropriate. The selection of the appropriate module is based on expressive language level rather than chronological age or cognitive ability, ensuring that the assessment tasks are accessible and appropriate for the individual being assessed.

Module 4, the focus of adult assessment, consists of a series of structured activities and conversations designed to provide opportunities for observation of social communication and interaction. The administration follows a standardized protocol while allowing some flexibility to maintain a natural flow of interaction. The activities include:

1. **Conversation and reporting**: Engaging in conversation about work, school, friends, and emotions, providing opportunities to observe reciprocal conversation skills, topic maintenance, and sharing of information
2. **Telling a story from a book**: Narrating a story from a picture book, allowing observation of narrative skills, perspective-taking, and integration of gesture with speech

3. **Description of a picture**: Describing a complex scene, providing opportunities to observe integration of elements into a coherent narrative
4. **Construction task**: Demonstrating how to build a simple structure, allowing observation of demonstration skills, coordination of verbal and non-verbal communication, and ability to take another's perspective
5. **Make-believe play**: Creating a simple story using objects, providing opportunities to observe imaginative abilities
6. **Joint interactive play**: Engaging in a cooperative activity, allowing observation of turn-taking, sharing enjoyment, and social reciprocity
7. **Conversation and reporting (emotions):** Discussing emotions and social relationships, providing opportunities to observe understanding and reporting of social-emotional experiences
8. **Break**: An unstructured period that allows observation of spontaneous social initiation and conversation
9. **Daily living**: Discussion of independence, responsibilities, and future plans, providing context for understanding adaptive functioning
10. **Friends, relationships, and marriage**: Conversation about social relationships, allowing observation of understanding of social relationships and their features
11. **Loneliness:** Discussion of emotions related to social connections, providing opportunities to observe emotional insight and reporting
12. **Creating a story**: Creating a narrative using objects, allowing observation of imagination and narrative skills

Throughout these activities, the examiner observes and codes specific behaviours relevant to autism diagnosis, including:

- Quality of social overtures and responses
- Amount and quality of reciprocal social communication
- Use of eye contact to regulate social interaction
- Facial expressions directed toward others
- Integration of verbal and non-verbal communication
- Insight into social relationships and emotions
- Use of descriptive, conventional, and instrumental gestures
- Stereotyped or idiosyncratic use of words or phrases
- Unusual sensory interests or mannerisms
- Excessive interest in unusual or highly specific topics or objects

- Compulsions or rituals

The administration time for Module 4 typically ranges from 45-60 minutes, though this can vary based on the individual's response style and engagement. Following administration, scoring requires an additional 15-30 minutes, making the total time commitment for a single ADOS-2 assessment approximately 60-90 minutes.

The scoring of the ADOS-2 involves rating observed behaviours on a scale of 0 (no evidence of abnormality related to autism), 1 (mild abnormality), 2 (moderate abnormality), or 3 (severe abnormality). These ratings are applied to specific items across two primary domains: **Social Affect (SA)** and **Restricted and Repetitive Behaviours (RRB)**. After completing all ratings, scores from selected items are summed to create algorithm scores for each domain, which are then combined to create a total score. This total score is compared to established cut-off values that indicate whether the individual's behaviours are consistent with autism, autism spectrum, or non-spectrum presentation.

The current ADOS-2 algorithm for Module 4 includes the following items:

Social Affect (SA) Domain:

- Unusual eye contact
- Facial expressions directed to examiner
- Empathy/comments on others' emotions
- Insight into typical social relationships
- Quality of social response
- Amount of reciprocal social communication
- Overall quality of rapport

Restricted and Repetitive Behaviours (RRB) Domain:

- Stereotyped/idiosyncratic use of words or phrases
- Unusual sensory interest in play material/person
- Hand, finger, and other complex mannerisms
- Excessive interest in or references to unusual or highly specific topics or objects or repetitive behaviours

It's important to note that the ADOS-2 algorithm focuses on a subset of the behaviours observed during administration, selected for their diagnostic specificity. However, clinically valuable information can be gleaned from all observations made during the assessment, even those not included in the formal algorithm.

While the ADOS-2 provides standardized scores and classifications, these should never be applied mechanistically in diagnostic decision-making. The ADOS-2 results represent one component of a comprehensive assessment and should be integrated with developmental history, self-report, informant report, and other observations to reach diagnostic conclusions. Several factors may influence ADOS-2 performance and should be considered in interpretation:

1. **State factors**: Anxiety, fatigue, medication effects, or current mood may influence presentation during the ADOS-2, potentially affecting scores
2. **Compensatory strategies**: Adults with autism, particularly those with higher cognitive abilities, may have developed sophisticated compensatory strategies that mask autism features in structured settings like the ADOS-2
3. **Gender**: The ADOS-2 may be less sensitive to female presentations of autism, which often involve more subtle social differences and sophisticated camouflaging
4. **Cultural factors**: Social communication norms vary across cultures, and the ADOS-2 was developed primarily in Western contexts, potentially affecting its cross-cultural validity
5. **Practice effects**: Individuals who have previously undergone autism assessment or who have researched autism extensively may be familiar with the types of tasks included and may consciously or unconsciously adapt their behaviour accordingly

The validity of the ADOS-2 for UK adult populations has been established through research studies, showing good sensitivity and specificity in discriminating between autism and non-autism presentations. However, like all standardized measures, its performance is not perfect, and both false positives and false negatives can occur. This reinforces the importance of comprehensive assessment rather than reliance on any single measure.

In UK clinical practice, the ADOS-2 is widely recognized as a key component of gold-standard assessment but is not universally implemented due to resource constraints and training limitations. NICE guidelines recommend consideration of autism-specific instruments as part of comprehensive assessment but do not mandate specific measures. Services should prioritize ensuring that at least some team members have ADOS-2 training, allowing for its use in complex or ambiguous cases even if resource constraints prevent its routine use with all referrals.

When properly administered and interpreted as part of a comprehensive assessment, the ADOS-2 provides valuable observational data that enhances diagnostic accuracy and contributes to a nuanced understanding of the individual's social communication profile. Its standardized nature allows for more consistent assessment across different clinicians and services, contributing to equity in diagnostic practices.

CHAPTER 10

ADI-R

(Autism Diagnostic Interview-Revised)

The **Autism Diagnostic Interview-Revised (ADI-R)** represents one of the most comprehensive and well-validated instruments for obtaining a detailed developmental history relevant to autism spectrum disorder. Developed by *Michael Rutter*, *Ann Le Couteur*, and *Catherine Lord*, the ADI-R provides a structured interview format for gathering information from parents or caregivers about an individual's developmental history and current behaviour. For adult autism assessment, the ADI-R offers a systematic approach to obtaining the developmental perspective that is essential for diagnosis but often challenging to access through self-report alone.

The primary purpose of the ADI-R is to collect detailed information about behaviours and developmental patterns that are relevant to autism diagnosis across three key domains: social interaction, communication, and restricted, repetitive, and stereotyped patterns of behaviour. The interview explores both historical development (particularly focusing on the age groups of 4-5 years, when autism features are often most clearly evident) and current behaviour. This developmental perspective is crucial for autism diagnosis, as autism is defined as a neurodevelopmental condition with early onset, even when recognition may occur much later in life.

Like the ADOS-2, formal training and certification are mandatory for administering the ADI-R in clinical practice. The complexity of the interview, the specific coding conventions, and the nuanced interpretation of responses require specialized training to ensure reliable and valid results. Formal ADI-R training typically involves:

1. A comprehensive clinical training workshop (typically 2-3 days) covering the theoretical background, interview techniques, coding conventions, and algorithm applications
2. Practice administrations with supervision and feedback

3. Demonstration of coding reliability compared to established standards
4. Ongoing maintenance of skills through regular use and refresher training

In the UK, ADI-R training is available through various providers, including university-based research centres and specialized training organizations. While representing a significant investment of time and resources, this training is essential for services aiming to provide comprehensive, evidence-based autism assessment. Using the ADI-R without proper training compromises the reliability and validity of the information obtained and would not meet standards for best practice.

The ADI-R is structured as a 93-item interview that systematically explores developmental history and current behaviour across multiple domains. The interview typically takes between 1.5 to 3 hours to complete, depending on the complexity of the individual's history and the informant's response style. This time investment reflects the comprehensive nature of the interview, which covers:

1. Early development, including pregnancy, birth, early milestones, and early concerns
2. Acquisition and loss of language and other skills
3. Language and communication functioning, including verbal and non-verbal communication
4. Social development and play, including peer relationships, social reciprocity, and imaginative play
5. Interests and behaviours, including restricted interests, routines, rituals, and sensory sensitivities
6. Clinically relevant behaviours such as aggression, self-injury, or overactivity
7. General behavioural concerns across development

For each area, the interviewer asks specific questions designed to elicit detailed examples of behaviours rather than general impressions or judgments. This focus on specific behavioural examples enhances the reliability of the information and reduces the influence of informant interpretation or bias. For instance, rather than asking if the person had unusual interests, the interviewer might ask about specific interests, their intensity, how much time was spent on them, and whether they interfered with other activities or social interactions.

The scoring of the ADI-R involves coding responses on a scale of 0 (behaviour not present), 1 (behaviour present but not sufficiently severe or frequent to meet criteria), 2 (definite abnormal behaviour of the type specified), or 3 (extreme severity of the specified behaviour). Certain items also include a code of 7 for definite abnormality in the general area of the coding, but not of the type specified in the item, or 8 for "not applicable." Following completion of all ratings, scores from selected items are used in diagnostic algorithms that indicate whether the pattern of historical development is consistent with autism.

One particular challenge in adult assessment is the historical recall required for accurate completion of the ADI-R. Parents or caregivers are asked to recall specific behaviours from when the individual was 4-5 years old, which may be several decades in the past for older adults. This retrospective recall introduces potential for various biases:

1. Memory decay: Simple forgetting of specific behaviours or developmental patterns over time
2. Reconstruction bias: Current knowledge of the individual's diagnosis or difficulties may influence recollection of early behaviours
3. Recall bias: More salient or unusual behaviours may be better remembered than typical development
4. Contrast effects: Early development may be recalled as more or less typical in contrast to later development

To mitigate these recall challenges, the skilled ADI-R interviewer employs several strategies:

1. Anchoring questions to specific developmental periods or life events (e.g., "Around the time he started school..." or "During the year you lived in Manchester...")
2. Asking for specific examples rather than general impressions
3. Using prompts to elicit detailed descriptions of behaviours
4. Cross-checking information against any available contemporaneous records such as school reports, home videos, or photographs
5. Acknowledging uncertainty and coding conservatively when recall is limited

Another significant challenge in adult assessment is the availability of informants who knew the individual during childhood. Parents may be deceased or otherwise unavailable, particularly for older adults seeking diagnosis. In such cases, creative approaches to gathering developmental information become necessary:

1. Interviewing siblings, extended family members, or longtime family friends who knew the person during childhood
2. Adapting the ADI-R for use with informants who had less consistent contact with the individual

3. Using any available historical records, such as school reports, childhood medical records, or family photographs and videos
4. Acknowledging limitations in historical information and placing greater emphasis on current presentation and consistent patterns across the lifespan

When parents are available for interview, they often provide invaluable insights that the individual themselves may not be able to report. Parents can describe behaviours that were present before the individual developed self-awareness or compensatory strategies, provide objective observations of social interactions and relationships, and identify patterns of behaviour that have remained consistent throughout development. This parental perspective often reveals autism features that may be masked in the individual's current presentation or self-report.

However, it's important to recognize that parental reports have their own limitations. Parents may have their own neurodevelopmental differences that affect their perceptions of typical versus atypical behaviour. Family dynamics and relationships may influence reporting, with some parents minimizing difficulties out of protective instincts or concern about stigma, while others may emphasize challenges in seeking support. Additionally, parents' understanding of autism may be limited or based on stereotypical presentations, affecting their recognition of relevant behaviours.

In UK clinical practice, the ADI-R is considered part of gold-standard assessment but is not universally implemented due to resource constraints, training limitations, and the practical challenges of interviewing informants for adult assessments. NICE guidelines recommend comprehensive developmental history as part of autism assessment but do not mandate specific instruments. Services should consider the ADI-R for complex cases or when diagnostic clarity is particularly challenging, even if resource constraints prevent its routine use with all referrals.

When the full ADI-R cannot be administered due to time constraints or limited informant availability, clinicians may adapt the approach by focusing on key items most relevant to diagnosis while maintaining the structured, example-focused interview style. While not providing the standardized scores of the full instrument, this adapted approach still yields valuable developmental information to complement current observations.

The integration of ADI-R findings with other assessment information requires clinical judgment and thoughtful consideration of potential discrepancies. Informant reports may sometimes conflict with the individual's self-report or with direct observations +during the ADOS-2. Such discrepancies do not invalidate either source but rather highlight the context-dependent nature of autism features and the different perspectives that various informants bring. The skilled clinician considers these multiple perspectives to develop a comprehensive understanding of the individual's developmental trajectory and current presentation.

CHAPTER 11

Additional Assessment Tools for Adults

Beyond the gold-standard ADOS-2 and ADI-R, a range of additional assessment tools is available for evaluating autism features in adults. These instruments vary in their format, focus, administration time, and psychometric properties, offering clinicians flexibility in selecting measures appropriate to the specific assessment context and individual being assessed. While none of these tools should be used in isolation for diagnostic purposes, they provide valuable complementary information as part of a comprehensive assessment approach.

The **Autism Spectrum Quotient (AQ)**, developed by Simon Baron-Cohen and his colleagues at the University of Cambridge, is one of the most widely used self-report measures for assessing autistic traits in adults with average or above-average intellectual ability. The standard version consists of 50 statements covering five domains: social skills, attention switching, attention to detail, communication, and imagination. Respondents rate their agreement with each statement on a 4-point scale (definitely agree, slightly agree, slightly disagree, definitely disagree), with responses scored as 0 or 1 depending on the direction of the trait. Total scores range from 0 to 50, with higher scores indicating more autistic traits. A score of 32 or above has been suggested as a cut-off indicating potential ASD in clinical samples, though this threshold should not be applied mechanistically for diagnostic purposes.

The AQ has demonstrated good psychometric properties, including test-retest reliability and internal consistency. It has been translated into numerous languages and has UK-specific validation, making it particularly appropriate for use in UK clinical settings. Shorter versions, including a 10-item screening version (AQ-10), have been developed for more rapid screening, though these have lower sensitivity and specificity than the full instrument.

The strengths of the AQ include its accessibility, ease of administration, and relatively good discrimination between autism and non-autism in adult populations without intellectual disabilities. However, several limitations should be considered: the AQ relies on self-awareness and insight, which may be variable in autism; it may be less sensitive to female presentations of autism; and scores may be elevated in other conditions with social difficulties, such as social anxiety disorder or schizoid personality disorder. Despite these limitations, the AQ provides a useful initial screening tool and a structured way to gather the individual's own perspective on traits related to autism.

Ritvo Autism Asperger Diagnostic Scale–Revised (RAADS-R)

The **Ritvo Autism Asperger Diagnostic Scale-Revised (RAADS-R)** is an 80-item self-report measure designed specifically for diagnosing autism in adults. The RAADS-R was developed to address the need for a self-report measure that incorporated DSM-IV criteria for autism and Asperger's syndrome while being appropriate for adults who may have more subtle presentations. The instrument assesses four domains: **social relatedness, circumscribed interests, language**, and **sensory-motor**. Unlike the AQ, the RAADS-R includes a temporal dimension, asking respondents to indicate whether each behaviour was true "now and when I was young," "only now," "only when I was younger than 16," or "never true." This temporal aspect provides valuable information about developmental trajectory and potential adaptations over time.

The RAADS-R has demonstrated good psychometric properties, including high sensitivity (97%) and specificity (100%) in distinguishing between adults with and without autism in the original validation studies. A total score of 65 or higher has been suggested as a cut-off indicating likely autism, though this should be interpreted in the context of the overall assessment.

The primary strengths of the RAADS-R include its focus on the developmental course of symptoms and its specific design for adult assessment. Its limitations parallel those of other self-report measures, including reliance on self-awareness and potential overlap with other conditions. Additionally, the length of the instrument (80 items) may be challenging for individuals with attention difficulties or executive functioning challenges, though a shorter 14-item version (RAADS-14) has been developed for screening purposes.

The Social Responsiveness Scale–2 (SRS-2): An Observer-Rated Measure of Social Impairment

The **Social Responsiveness Scale-2 (SRS-2)** provides a dimensional measure of social impairment associated with autism. Unlike the AQ and RAADS-R, which were developed primarily as self-report measures, the SRS-2 was designed as an observer-rated measure to be completed by someone who knows the individual well, such as a parent, partner, or close friend. The adult version consists of 65 items covering **social awareness, social cognition, social communication,**

social motivation, and **restricted interests/repetitive behaviours**. Responses are rated on a 4-point scale from "not true" to "almost always true," with total T-scores providing an indication of the severity of social impairment.

The SRS-2 has strong psychometric properties and provides standardized T-scores based on large normative samples, allowing comparison to age and gender-matched peers. It is particularly valuable for quantifying the severity of social difficulties across a continuum, rather than simply providing a binary indication of autism/non-autism. This dimensional approach aligns well with current conceptualizations of autism as a spectrum condition.

The observer-rated nature of the SRS-2 provides an important complementary perspective to self-report, potentially capturing aspects of social functioning that the individual may not recognize. However, this also introduces potential reporter bias, and ratings may be influenced by the nature and context of the relationship between the individual and the rater. Additionally, elevated scores on the SRS-2 may reflect social difficulties associated with conditions other than autism.

Adult Asperger Assessment (AAA)

The **Adult Asperger Assessment (AAA)** combines the AQ with the Empathy Quotient (EQ) to provide a more comprehensive assessment of autistic traits and empathy. Developed by Simon Baron-Cohen and his colleagues, the AAA was designed specifically for diagnosing Asperger syndrome (now incorporated within the broader autism spectrum disorder diagnosis) in adults with average or above-average intelligence. The AAA algorithm converts AQ and EQ scores into a diagnostic format aligned with DSM-IV and ICD-10 criteria, providing a structured approach to diagnostic decision-making based on self-report.

The AAA has the advantage of specifically addressing empathy, which is a key aspect of social-cognitive functioning in autism that may not be fully captured by other instruments. However, it shares the limitations of other self-report measures and may not fully capture the more subtle presentations of autism, particularly in women. Additionally, the diagnostic algorithm was developed for Asperger syndrome specifically and may need adaptation for use with the broader autism spectrum disorder category in current diagnostic systems.

Developmental, Dimensional and Diagnostic Interview (3Di)

The **Developmental, Dimensional and Diagnostic Interview (3Di)** represents an alternative to the ADI-R for obtaining developmental history relevant to autism diagnosis. The 3Di is a computerized, semi-structured interview designed to be administered to parents or caregivers. The adult version has been adapted to address the challenges of retrospective reporting for adult diagnosis. Like the ADI-R, the 3Di systematically explores developmental history across domains relevant to autism diagnosis, but its computerized format allows for more flexible administration and automatic algorithm scoring.

The 3Di has demonstrated good agreement with the ADI-R while potentially offering advantages in terms of administration time and accessibility. Its computerized format may enhance standardization across different interviewers and settings. However, it shares the challenges of all developmental history interviews regarding retrospective recall and informant availability for adult assessment.

Several additional questionnaires may provide valuable information about specific aspects of autism-related functioning:

The **Sensory Profile (Adult version)** assesses sensory processing patterns across multiple sensory domains, providing detailed information about sensory sensitivities, seeking behaviours, and avoidance that may inform understanding of restricted and repetitive behaviours as well as daily functioning challenges.

The **Reading the Mind in the Eyes Test** evaluates emotion recognition from eye expressions, providing a measure of one aspect of social cognition that is often affected in autism.

The **Friendship Questionnaire** assesses the quality and nature of friendships and social relationships, providing information about social functioning that may complement other measures.

Executive functioning questionnaires, such as the **Behaviour Rating Inventory of Executive Function (BRIEF-A)**, may identify patterns of executive functioning strengths and challenges that commonly co-occur with autism and impact daily functioning.

When selecting among these various instruments, several considerations should guide clinical decision-making:

1. **Purpose of assessment**: Different measures may be more appropriate depending on whether the primary goal is screening, comprehensive diagnostic assessment, or detailed profiling of strengths and challenges for support planning.
2. **Available informants**: The selection of measures should consider whether reliable informants are available for developmental history or current observational reports.

3. **Cognitive and language abilities**: Measures should be selected that are appropriate for the individual's cognitive and language levels, as many standard instruments assume average intellectual ability and good reading comprehension.
4. **Time constraints**: Pragmatic considerations regarding assessment time may influence the selection of briefer versus more comprehensive measures.
5. **Psychometric properties**: Preference should be given to measures with established reliability, validity, and normative data for the UK adult population when available.

It is crucial to emphasize that none of these instruments should be used in isolation for diagnostic purposes. Each provides a partial view of the complex presentation of autism, and all have limitations in terms of sensitivity, specificity, and breadth of coverage. A multi-method assessment approach that integrates information from multiple sources and perspectives is essential for accurate diagnosis and comprehensive understanding of the individual's profile.

In UK clinical practice, access to these various instruments may be influenced by resource constraints, training requirements, and service protocols. While NICE guidelines do not mandate specific instruments, they emphasize the importance of comprehensive assessment using structured, validated approaches. Services should develop assessment protocols that incorporate a range of complementary measures while recognizing the practical limitations of time and resources.

CHAPTER 12

Assessment of Social Communication & Interaction

Social communication and interaction difficulties represent one of the two core diagnostic domains for autism spectrum disorder. A comprehensive assessment must thoroughly examine this domain, capturing both the obvious and subtle manifestations of social communication differences that characterize autism. This assessment requires careful observation across multiple contexts, structured assessment tasks, and detailed exploration of developmental history and current functioning through clinical interview.

Reciprocal conversation represents a complex social skill that many adults with autism find challenging, even when they have strong language abilities. Assessment of conversational skills should examine multiple components:

Turn-taking in conversation involves the balanced exchange of speaker and listener roles. Adults with autism may demonstrate various differences in turn-taking, including dominating conversation with monologues, having difficulty initiating conversational turns, or showing unusual patterns of interruption or delayed responses. The clinician should observe the natural flow of conversation throughout the assessment, noting whether the individual spontaneously asks questions of others, how they respond when asked questions, and whether they leave appropriate pauses for others to speak. It's important to distinguish between difficulties with the social understanding of turn-taking conventions and other factors that might affect conversational flow, such as anxiety, executive functioning challenges affecting response inhibition, or cultural differences in conversational style.

Topic maintenance involves the ability to sustain a coherent thread of conversation, introducing related points and following others' topic shifts appropriately. Adults with autism may show several patterns of difference in this area: some may adhere rigidly to preferred topics, repeatedly returning to these despite others' attempts to shift the conversation; others may make tangential comments that reflect associative rather than logical connections between ideas;

still others may shift topics abruptly without signalling the change or establishing the relevance of the new topic. Assessment should note the individual's flexibility in topic shifts, relevance of contributions, and awareness of others' interest in the topic.

Responding to social cues requires the ability to recognize and adapt to subtle signals in conversation, such as others' body language indicating boredom, confusion, or desire to speak. Individuals with autism may miss these cues or have difficulty integrating them into their conversational regulation in real time. The assessment should include observation of how the individual responds to the examiner's social signals, such as looking at their watch, shifting posture, or using facial expressions indicating confusion or interest. Structured opportunities to observe these responses can be created by deliberately introducing such cues during conversation.

Nonverbal communication differences represent another key aspect of social communication in autism. Unlike verbal language, which may be a relative strength for many adults with autism without intellectual disabilities, nonverbal communication often remains challenging even for those with strong compensation strategies. Assessment should examine several components:

Eye contact should be assessed in terms of both quantity and quality. Quantitative aspects include the frequency and duration of eye contact, while qualitative aspects include the coordination of eye contact with speech, its modulation based on conversational content, and its use for different communicative functions (e.g., greeting, checking understanding, emphasizing points). Many adults with autism report that they have learned to make deliberate eye contact in professional or formal situations, so assessment should consider whether eye contact appears natural or effortful, and whether it varies across different conversational contexts within the assessment. Cultural differences in eye contact norms should also be considered, as expectations vary significantly across cultural contexts.

Facial expressions should be examined for their range, appropriateness to context, integration with verbal content, and subtlety. Adults with autism may show limited facial expressiveness (often described as a "flat affect"), exaggerated expressions that don't match the emotional content of the conversation, or brief expressions that aren't sustained naturally throughout the interaction. Assessment should note whether expressions appear spontaneous or rehearsed, whether they match the emotional content being discussed, and whether subtle expressions (such as brief micro expressions) are present. The individual's ability to modulate expressions based on social context is particularly informative, as many adults with autism have learned to produce basic expressions but may struggle with the nuanced social modulation of expression intensity.

Gestures encompass a range of hand and body movements that accompany and enhance verbal communication. These include descriptive gestures that illustrate verbal content (e.g., showing the size or shape of something), conventional gestures that replace words (e.g., waving goodbye), and emphatic gestures that accent speech. Adults with autism may use fewer gestures overall, employ unusual or idiosyncratic gestures, or show poor integration of gestures with speech, such that gestures occur after or disconnected from the related verbal content. Assessment should note both the frequency and quality of different types of gestures, considering whether they enhance communication effectively and appear natural rather than rehearsed.

Body language includes aspects of physical positioning and movement such as orientation toward conversation partners, physical proximity, posture, and general motor coordination during social interaction. Individuals with autism may stand too close or too far from others, position themselves at unusual angles during conversation, or show limited adaptation of posture based on social context. The assessment should observe how the individual positions themselves relative to others, how they adjust their posture and position during different activities, and whether their overall physical presentation facilitates or hinders social connection.

Emotional reciprocity involves the mutual sharing and responding to emotional states between interaction partners. This includes recognizing others' emotions, responding appropriately to their emotional cues, and sharing one's own emotional experiences in socially modulated ways. Adults with autism may struggle with accurately identifying others' emotions, particularly from subtle or complex cues. They may respond in ways that appear unexpected or mismatched to others' emotional states, such as providing logical solutions when emotional support is sought, or not adjusting their behaviour in response to others' distress or enthusiasm. Assessment should include discussion of emotional topics and observation of how the individual recognizes, interprets, and responds to the examiner's emotional expressions throughout the assessment.

Relationships assessment explores both the historical development and current state of the individual's social connections. This includes examining the quantity and quality of friendships throughout development, understanding of different relationship types and their associated social rules, and ability to form and maintain relationships across contexts. Adults with autism often report distinctive relationship patterns, such as having few but intense friendships, struggling with the transition from acquaintance to friend, or finding relationships more successful when organized around shared special interests or structured activities. Assessment should explore not only whether the individual has relationships but also their quality, reciprocity, and the individual's understanding of their dynamics. This includes understanding of unstated social rules, capacity for compromise, and navigation of conflict within relationships.

Social cognition refers to the mental processes involved in understanding and navigating the social world. This includes theory of mind (the ability to understand that others have mental states different from one's own), perspective-taking, understanding of social hierarchies and contexts, and interpretation of ambiguous social situations. Assessment of social cognition may include both formal measures, such as the Reading the Mind in the Eyes Test or theory of mind vignettes, and informal exploration through clinical interview. Questions that probe social understanding might include asking the individual to explain why a character in a story acted as they did, how they would interpret ambiguous social scenarios, or how they understand different types of humour (particularly sarcasm, irony, or jokes that require understanding others' perspectives).

When assessing social communication and interaction, several methodological considerations are important:

1. Create multiple contexts for observation, as social communication may vary significantly based on topic, structure, and comfort level. Include both structured and unstructured interactions, conversations about factual and emotional topics, and if possible, observations in different physical settings.
2. Consider compensatory strategies that may mask underlying differences. Many adults with autism, particularly those diagnosed later in life, have developed sophisticated compensation strategies that may make social difficulties less apparent in brief or structured interactions. These strategies often require considerable cognitive effort and may break down under stress, fatigue, or in novel social situations.
3. Explore developmental changes in social communication. Many adults report that their social understanding has improved with age through explicit learning, while the effort required for social interaction may have increased due to the growing complexity of adult social contexts.
4. Distinguish between social capacity and social motivation. Some individuals with autism have limited interest in social interaction despite adequate social skills, while others have strong social motivation but significant difficulties with social understanding and execution. This distinction has important implications for support planning.

5. Assess social communication in relation to the individual's overall cognitive profile, as strengths in verbal reasoning, memory, or logical analysis may be used to compensate for intuitive social difficulties.

The assessment of social communication and interaction should ultimately aim not simply to document deficits but to understand the individual's unique social style, strengths, challenges, and adaptation strategies. This nuanced understanding forms the foundation for meaningful support recommendations that respect the individual's social preferences while addressing areas where social differences cause distress or functional impairment.

CHAPTER 13

Detailed Assessment of Nonverbal Communication

Nonverbal communication comprises a complex system of behaviours that accompany, enhance, modify, or replace verbal language in social interaction. While verbal communication tends to convey explicit content, nonverbal communication often transmits emotional states, social attitudes, and relationship dynamics. For many adults with autism, nonverbal communication represents an area of significant challenge, even when verbal language skills are strong. A thorough assessment of nonverbal communication is therefore essential to understanding an individual's social communication profile and identifying areas where support might be beneficial.

Eye contact serves multiple functions in social communication: it signals attention and interest, regulates conversational turn-taking, emphasizes important points, and provides feedback on the listener's understanding and emotional response. The assessment of eye contact should go beyond simply noting its presence or absence to examine patterns that might indicate autism-related differences.

Various eye contact patterns may be observed in adults with autism. Some individuals may make very little or no eye contact, consistently looking away from the conversation partner's face. Others may make brief or fleeting eye contact, making momentary eye contact before quickly looking away. Some may demonstrate fixed or staring eye contact, maintaining gaze for uncomfortably long periods without the typical small breaks that characterize neurotypical eye contact patterns. Still others may show context-inappropriate eye contact, such as looking away during moments when eye contact would typically be expected (e.g., greetings or important points in conversation) or making intense eye contact during moments when gaze would typically be averted (e.g., during brief silences or when discussing sensitive topics).

The modulation of eye contact based on emotional content or social demands represents a particularly sophisticated aspect of nonverbal communication. Neurotypical individuals typically increase eye contact when listening and during emotionally connecting moments, while slightly reducing eye contact when speaking or processing complex information. They also adjust eye contact based on relationship dynamics, social hierarchy, and cultural context. Adults with autism may show less variation in eye contact across these different contexts, maintaining a more consistent pattern regardless of the emotional content or social demands of the interaction.

When assessing eye contact, clinicians should observe patterns throughout the assessment rather than at isolated moments, as eye contact may fluctuate based on anxiety, topic interest, and familiarity with the examiner. It's also important to distinguish between difficulties with eye contact that reflect autism-related differences in social communication and those that might be explained by other factors such as social anxiety, cultural norms, or trauma history. Direct questioning about the subjective experience of eye contact can provide valuable insights, as many adults with autism report that eye contact feels uncomfortable, overwhelming, or distracting, making it difficult to simultaneously maintain eye contact and process conversation.

Facial expressiveness represents another critical component of nonverbal communication. Facial expressions communicate emotional states, reactions to others' comments, interest level, and engagement in the interaction. The assessment of facial expressiveness should examine several dimensions:

The range of facial expressions includes the variety of distinct expressions the individual displays throughout the assessment. Adults with autism may show a limited range of expressions, with some emotions rarely or never reflected in their facial expressions despite being verbally reported. Assessment should note which emotions are expressed facially and which seem to be absent from the individual's expressive repertoire.

The appropriateness of facial expressions to content involves the match between the individual's expressions and the emotional tone of the conversation. Some adults with autism may show expressions that seem incongruent with the content being discussed, such as smiling while describing sad events or maintaining a neutral expression during emotionally charged topics. Others may show appropriate expressions but with unusual timing, such as delayed emotional reactions that occur after the relevant moment has passed in conversation.

The **subtlety of facial expressions** refers to the gradations of intensity and the presence of brief micro expressions that typically occur during social interaction. Adults with autism may show less nuanced expressions, with more all-or-nothing displays rather than the subtle gradations that characterize typical emotional expression. They may also show fewer of the brief micro expressions that signal momentary reactions to conversational content.

When assessing facial expressiveness, it's important to recognize potential compensatory strategies. Many adults with autism report consciously working to produce appropriate facial expressions in social situations, which may result in expressions that are technically correct but appear somewhat mechanical or exaggerated. These learned expressions may be distinguished from spontaneous expressions by their timing, maintenance, and integration with other aspects of communication.

Gesture use encompasses a rich vocabulary of hand and body movements that accompany speech, adding emphasis, clarity, and emotional tone to verbal communication. The assessment of gesture should examine different types of gestures and their integration with verbal communication:

Descriptive gestures illustrate aspects of verbal content, such as showing the size or shape of an object, demonstrating an action, or indicating direction. These iconic gestures enhance the listener's understanding by providing visual representation of concepts being discussed. Adults with autism may use fewer descriptive gestures overall or may use them in less integrated ways, such as gesturing after completing the related verbal description rather than simultaneously.

Conventional gestures are culturally standardized movements that have specific meanings, such as waving goodbye, nodding for yes, or giving a thumbs-up. These gestures can sometimes replace words entirely in communication. Some adults with autism may use conventional gestures appropriately but in a way that appears somewhat learned or mechanical rather than naturally integrated into communication.

Emphatic gestures accompany speech to add emphasis, express emotion, or regulate the pace and flow of conversation. These gestures don't convey specific semantic content but rather enhance the delivery of the message. Adults with autism often show reduced use of emphatic gestures, contributing to an overall impression of less animated or engaging communication style.

The integration of gestures with verbal communication is particularly important to assess. Typically developing individuals seamlessly coordinate their gestures with the related verbal content, with the gesture either slightly preceding or occurring simultaneously with the words it relates to. Adults with autism may show poor temporal synchronization, with gestures occurring after the related words or seeming disconnected from the verbal flow. This poor integration can make communication less clear and engaging, even when the individual is using appropriate types of gestures.

Assessment should note not only the frequency and types of gestures used but also their quality, timing, and natural integration into the overall communication style. It's also important to consider cultural variations in gesture use, as the frequency and style of gesturing varies significantly across different cultural contexts.

Prosody refers to the rhythm, stress, and intonation patterns of speech, which convey emotional tone, emphasis, and sometimes grammatical distinctions (such as the difference between a statement and a question). Prosodic differences are common in autism and can significantly impact how communication is perceived by others. Assessment should examine:

- Rhythm and rate of speech, noting whether it flows naturally or shows unusual patterns such as a consistently monotone delivery, exaggerated variations, or odd timing of pauses.
- Stress patterns, including whether emphasis is placed on appropriate words to convey meaning and whether this emphasis is communicated through typical combinations of volume, pitch, and timing.
- Intonation, particularly the appropriate rising and falling patterns that signal questions, statements, and emotional tone.
- Volume regulation, including whether the individual modulates their volume appropriately for the social context and conversational content.

Prosodic differences in autism might include monotone speech (limited variation in pitch and emphasis), exaggerated or sing-song patterns, unusual stress on typically emphasized words or syllables, or volume that doesn't adjust appropriately to the social context. Some individuals may show adequate prosody when reading prepared material but revert to atypical patterns in spontaneous speech, highlighting the importance of assessing prosody across different communication contexts.

Personal space awareness involves understanding and respecting cultural and social norms regarding physical proximity during interaction. This aspect of nonverbal communication reflects an implicit understanding of social boundaries that many adults with autism find challenging. Assessment should observe:

The individual's positioning relative to others during natural movements within the assessment session, adjustments to physical distance based on the nature of the interaction and relationship, and recognition of others' cues regarding comfortable distance Cultural considerations regarding typical proximity patterns

Adults with autism may stand too close to others (uncomfortably invading personal space) or position themselves too far away for effective communication. They may also show less adaptation of distance based on the nature of the relationship or interaction, maintaining similar proximity patterns regardless of context. Some individuals may demonstrate appropriate distance but report that this is a learned behaviour rather than an intuitive understanding, requiring conscious monitoring in social situations.

When assessing nonverbal communication, several methodological considerations are important:

1. Observe behaviours across different contexts within the assessment, including casual conversation, structured tasks, emotional discussions, and transitions between activities. Nonverbal communication may vary based on the individual's comfort, interest, and familiarity with the type of interaction.
2. Consider potential compensatory strategies that may mask underlying differences. Many adults with autism have developed conscious techniques to manage aspects of nonverbal communication, such as deliberate eye contact or rehearsed facial expressions. These strategies may be identified by their somewhat mechanical quality, inconsistent implementation when the individual is focused on complex content, or the visible effort they require.
3. Distinguish between nonverbal communication differences that reflect autism and those that might be explained by other factors such as anxiety, cultural background, family communication patterns, or co-occurring conditions.
4. Gather the individual's own perspective on nonverbal communication through direct questioning. Many adults with autism can provide valuable insights into their experience of making eye contact, reading others' expressions, or managing physical proximity.
5. Where possible, obtain information about nonverbal communication in everyday settings outside the assessment context, as some individuals may demonstrate different patterns in familiar versus unfamiliar environments.

The assessment of nonverbal communication should ultimately aim to understand the individual's unique profile of strengths and challenges in this domain, identifying specific aspects that may contribute to social communication difficulties in daily life. This detailed understanding can inform targeted recommendations for support and accommodation, such as explicit instruction in reading nonverbal cues, environmental modifications to reduce the processing demands of nonverbal communication, or education for family members and colleagues about the individual's nonverbal communication style.

CHAPTER 14

Assessment of Restricted & Repetitive Behaviours

Restricted and repetitive behaviours represent the second core diagnostic domain for autism spectrum disorder. This domain encompasses a diverse range of behaviours, interests, and activities that share qualities of repetition, rigidity, invariance, or intensity. While social communication differences are often more immediately apparent in clinical settings, a thorough assessment of restricted and repetitive behaviours is essential for accurate diagnosis and comprehensive understanding of the individual's autism presentation. This domain manifests in various ways across development and may be expressed differently in adults compared to children, requiring careful and nuanced assessment approaches.

Special interests represent one of the most distinctive and clinically significant manifestations of the restricted and repetitive behaviour domain in adults with autism, particularly those without intellectual disabilities. These interests differ from typical hobbies or professional interests in several key dimensions that should be assessed:

Intensity refers to the depth of engagement with the interest, including the amount of time devoted to it, the level of detailed knowledge acquired, and the emotional investment in the topic. Adults with autism often develop exceptional expertise in their areas of interest, accumulating vast amounts of information and dedicating substantial time to pursuing the interest. Assessment should explore not only what topics interest the individual but also how they engage with these topics, including the time spent, information collected, and priority given to the interest relative to other life activities.

Persistence describes the duration of interests over time. While many people cycle through different hobbies and interests throughout life, individuals with autism often maintain their special interests for extended periods, sometimes throughout the lifespan. Alternatively, some may show a pattern of serially intense interests, moving from one all-consuming focus to another. The assessment should explore the historical pattern of interests, noting their longevity and whether they tend to be maintained alongside new interests or replaced by them.

Unusual focus describes the nature of the interest itself or the specific aspect that captivates the individual. Some adults with autism are interested in topics that are unusual for their age, gender, or cultural context. Others may have interests in common topics but focus on particular aspects that are unusual, such as collecting detailed statistics about a sport rather than following teams or players, or memorizing transportation timetables rather than traveling to destinations. Assessment should note both the general topic area and the specific focus within it that engages the individual.

Interference with daily functioning represents an important clinical dimension that distinguishes special interests that may warrant diagnostic significance from those that represent typical passions or hobbies. Assessment should explore whether the interest takes precedence over essential activities such as self-care, sleep, work responsibilities, or maintaining relationships. Some adults with autism report difficulty disengaging from their interests to attend to other necessary activities, leading to practical challenges in daily life.

Social Sharing vs. Monologuing: Assessing Reciprocity in Communication

Social sharing versus monologuing reflects the way the individual communicates about their interests in social contexts. Typical interests are usually shared in a reciprocal manner, with awareness of the listener's interest level and knowledge. In contrast, adults with autism may engage in one-sided monologues about their interests, showing limited adaptation to the listener's verbal and nonverbal cues indicating boredom or lack of shared enthusiasm. Assessment should observe how the individual discusses their interests during the evaluation, noting whether they show awareness of the listener's engagement, adjust the level of detail based on the listener's knowledge, and recognize when to transition to other topics.

Routines and rituals encompass the need for consistency, predictability, and specific patterns in daily activities. These may manifest in various ways in adult life:

- **Need for predictability and sameness** may be observed in rigid daily schedules, consistent routines for specific activities, or distress when expected patterns are disrupted. Adults with autism may create highly structured daily routines that provide a sense of order and predictability, following the same sequence of activities each day or at specific times. Assessment should explore the individual's typical daily patterns, noting the degree of consistency maintained and whether this reflects preference or necessity for functioning.

- **Ritualized patterns** involve specific sequences or methods for completing activities that must be followed precisely. These might include particular orders for morning routines, specific approaches to organizing possessions, or ritualized ways of entering or navigating environments. Assessment should explore whether the individual has specific "rules" for how activities must be done, noting the rigidity of these patterns and their impact on daily functioning.
- **Response to change or interruption** provides crucial clinical information about the function and impact of routines and rituals. Adults with autism may experience varying levels of distress when routines are disrupted, ranging from mild irritation to significant anxiety or behavioural disturbance. Assessment should explore specific examples of how the individual responds when expected routines cannot be followed, plans change unexpectedly, or rituals are interrupted. This includes noting both emotional responses (anxiety, anger, shutdown) and behavioural adaptations (withdrawal, insistence on completing the routine, difficulty transitioning to alternative activities).
- **Cognitive flexibility**, the ability to shift between different thoughts, actions, or approaches, is often affected in autism and relates closely to routines and rituals. Assessment may include formal cognitive measures of set-shifting abilities or clinical exploration of how easily the individual can adapt their thinking and behaviour when circumstances change. Limited cognitive flexibility may manifest as difficulty generating alternative solutions to problems, seeing situations from multiple perspectives, or adapting established approaches when they no longer work effectively.
- **Repetitive movement and sensory regulation**, often called stereotypies or self-stimulatory behaviours, include repetitive motor actions that appear to serve sensory or regulatory functions. While often more prominent in children or individuals with intellectual disabilities, many adults with autism without intellectual disabilities also experience these movements, though they may have developed strategies to limit them in public settings.

Assessment should explore several aspects:

1. Hand and finger mannerisms may include hand-flapping, finger-flicking, complex finger movements, or unusual hand posturing. These movements often occur during emotional states such as excitement, anxiety, or deep concentration.

2. Whole body movements might include rocking, swaying, pacing in fixed patterns, spinning, or bouncing. These larger movements may be more likely to occur in private settings where social judgment is not a concern.

Context and triggers for repetitive movements provide important clinical information about their function. Assessment should explore when these behaviours typically occur, noting whether they are associated with particular emotional states, sensory environments, or activities. Many adults report that repetitive movements increase during stress or intense focus, or when they are alone and don't need to suppress them for social reasons.

Efforts to control repetitive movements in public settings should be explored, as many adults with autism describe consciously suppressing these behaviours in professional or social contexts, often at the cost of increased anxiety or mental effort. This suppression may contribute to the "masking" of autism features that often leads to delayed diagnosis, particularly in women.

Sensory sensitivities represent a clinically significant aspect of the restricted and repetitive behaviour domain that has gained increased recognition in current diagnostic frameworks. These sensory differences may manifest as either hypersensitivity (over-responsiveness) or hyposensitivity (under-responsiveness) across different sensory modalities, and often have substantial impacts on daily functioning.

Assessment should explore:

Hypersensitivity across sensory domains, including sensitivity to sounds (especially background noise, specific frequencies, or unpredictable sounds), lights (particularly fluorescent lighting or bright sunlight), tactile sensations (clothing textures, light touch, temperature), tastes (limited food preferences due to taste or texture sensitivities), smells (strong reactions to odours others may not notice), and vestibular or proprioceptive input (discomfort with certain movements or positions).

Hyposensitivity may manifest as reduced awareness of sensory input, such as diminished response to pain or temperature, seeking intense sensory experiences, or difficulty recognizing internal bodily sensations such as hunger or fatigue.

Unusual sensory interests involve fascination with or craving for specific sensory experiences, such as visual examination of light patterns, listening to particular sounds repeatedly, or seeking specific tactile sensations. These interests often have a repetitive quality and may serve regulatory functions.

Impact on daily functioning should be carefully assessed, as sensory sensitivities can significantly affect participation in work, education, social activities, and independent living. Common impacts include difficulty working in noisy or bright environments, challenges with public transportation due to sensory overload, limited food choices affecting social dining, or avoidance of crowded places due to tactile or auditory sensitivities.

Sensory adaptation strategies should be explored, as many adults with autism develop sophisticated approaches to managing their sensory environments, such as using noise-cancelling headphones, sunglasses, specific clothing choices, or careful environmental modifications at home and work. These adaptations may significantly reduce the observable impact of sensory sensitivities while not eliminating the underlying differences.

Rule-based behaviour involves rigid adherence to rules, systems, or principles, often extending beyond situations where such adherence is necessary or expected. This aspect of restricted and repetitive behaviours may manifest in various ways in adults:

Literal interpretation and application of rules, even when flexibility would be socially appropriate or pragmatically beneficial. Adults with autism may adhere strictly to workplace policies, social conventions, or agreed-upon plans, showing distress or confusion when others apply rules more flexibly.

Creation of personal rule systems to navigate complex or ambiguous situations. Some adults with autism develop elaborate personal rules for social interaction, decision-making, or daily activities as a way of creating predictability and structure in inherently variable situations.

Moral rigidity and justice orientation, with strong reactions to perceived unfairness or rule violations by others. Many adults with autism report intense emotional responses when rules are not followed or when exceptions are made that seem inconsistent with established principles.

Assessment of rule-based behaviour should explore the individual's approach to rules in various contexts, their flexibility in rule application, and their emotional and behavioural responses when rules are broken or changed. This exploration should distinguish between adherence to rules based on social or moral principles (which may reflect positive values) and rigid rule-following that creates functional difficulties or interpersonal challenges.

When assessing restricted and repetitive behaviours in adults, several methodological considerations are important:

1. Combine direct observation with self-report and collateral information, as some restricted and repetitive behaviours may be deliberately suppressed

in assessment settings or may occur primarily in specific contexts not observable during evaluation.

2. Consider developmental changes in expression, as many adults with autism report that their restricted and repetitive behaviours have evolved over time, often becoming less overtly apparent but maintaining similar underlying functions and qualities.
3. Explore the subjective experience and function of these behaviours, as many adults with autism can provide valuable insights into why certain routines, movements, or sensory experiences are important to them and what happens when they cannot engage in them.
4. Distinguish between restricted and repetitive behaviours that cause distress or functional impairment and those that represent differences that may be neutral or even adaptive in certain contexts.
5. Consider how these behaviours interact with environmental demands and support, as the impact of restricted and repetitive behaviours often depends significantly on the degree of accommodation in the individual's living and working environments.

The assessment of restricted and repetitive behaviours should ultimately aim to understand not only their presence and manifestation but also their function, impact, and meaning for the individual. This understanding can inform recommendations for environmental adaptations, coping strategies, and supports that respect the individual's needs for predictability and sensory comfort while addressing aspects that may cause distress or limit functioning.

CHAPTER 15
Sensory Assessment in Detail

Sensory processing differences represent a clinically significant aspect of autism that has gained increased recognition in current diagnostic frameworks. While historically considered a secondary feature, sensory sensitivities are now explicitly included in diagnostic criteria for autism spectrum disorder, acknowledging their prevalence and impact on daily functioning. For many adults with autism, sensory differences may cause more significant distress and functional impairment than social communication challenges, making thorough sensory assessment an essential component of the diagnostic process.

Sensory processing encompasses the ways in which the nervous system receives, organizes, and responds to sensory information from the environment and from within the body. Differences in sensory processing may manifest as hypersensitivity (over-responsiveness to sensory input), hyposensitivity (under-responsiveness to sensory input), or sensory seeking (craving or fascination with certain sensory experiences). These patterns can occur across any sensory domain and may vary within the same individual depending on context, stress level, and the specific nature of the sensory input.

Auditory processing differences are among the most commonly reported sensory challenges for adults with autism. Assessment should explore several dimensions of auditory sensitivity:

Hypersensitivity to specific sounds may include heightened awareness of and distress in response to particular auditory stimuli that others might not notice or find bothersome. Common triggers include high-pitched sounds (like alarms or whistles), certain mechanical noises (vacuum cleaners, hand dryers), chewing or mouth sounds, or specific speech characteristics. Assessment should identify specific sound sensitivities, the intensity of response, and the impact on daily functioning. For example, an individual might avoid using public restrooms due to fear of hand dryers or experience significant distress in restaurants due to background conversation and utensil noises.

Difficulty filtering background noise represents a particularly common and impactful auditory processing difference. Many adults with autism report challenges separating relevant auditory information (like a conversation partner's voice) from background sounds (such as café noise, air conditioning hum, or distant conversations). This difficulty can make social settings, open-plan offices, or public spaces extraordinarily challenging and exhausting. Assessment should explore the individual's experience in various auditory environments, noting settings that are particularly difficult and strategies developed to manage these challenges.

Unusual attention to subtle sounds involves heightened awareness of auditory stimuli that may go unnoticed by others. Some adults with autism report hearing electrical hums, distant conversations, or subtle environmental sounds that others in the same space do not perceive. This heightened perception may be distracting in environments where focus on other stimuli is required, such as workplaces or educational settings. Assessment should explore whether the individual experiences this heightened auditory awareness and how it impacts their concentration and comfort in different environments.

Auditory assessment should also note potential hyposensitivity or delayed processing of auditory information. Some individuals may have reduced response to certain sounds (like not responding to their name being called) or require additional processing time to comprehend auditory information, particularly complex or rapid speech. These patterns may coexist with hypersensitivities to other types of auditory input, creating complex profiles of auditory processing.

Visual processing differences can significantly impact comfort and functioning in various environments. Assessment should explore:

Hypersensitivity to lighting, particularly fluorescent lights, which many adults with autism report as causing visual discomfort, perceptual distortions, or headaches. Some individuals may be able to perceive the flickering of fluorescent lights that is imperceptible to most people, creating significant distress in environments where such lighting is common, such as offices, shops, or healthcare settings.

Sensitivity to movement within the visual field, where busy visual environments with multiple moving elements (such as crowded streets or shopping centres) may create overwhelming visual processing demands. Some adults report difficulty tracking relevant visual information when there is significant movement in their peripheral vision.

Preference for detail versus holistic processing reflects a cognitive pattern often associated with autism, where attention may be naturally drawn to specific details rather than the overall gestalt of visual information. This pattern may manifest as noticing small details that others miss or difficulty "seeing the forest for the trees" in visual processing. Assessment might explore whether the individual tends to notice specific elements of visual scenes before grasping the overall picture, or whether they find detailed visual search tasks relatively easy compared to processing complex visual scenes holistically.

Visual assessment should also consider potential visual strengths, such as enhanced pattern recognition, exceptional memory for visual details, or ability to detect visual irregularities. These visual processing strengths may be harnessed in educational or occupational settings while accommodating areas of visual sensitivity.

Tactile sensitivities are extremely common in autism and can have profound effects on daily activities such as dressing, eating, and physical contact with others. Assessment should explore:

Response to textures, particularly clothing textures, as many adults with autism report specific requirements for clothing based on tactile comfort. This might include needing to remove clothing tags, preferring certain fabric types, or being unable to tolerate seams, tight clothing, or certain fabric weights. These sensitivities may necessitate restricted clothing choices, affect professional presentation, or create distress when dress codes require uncomfortable items.

Response to touch from others, including sensitivity to light touch (which is often reported as more uncomfortable than firm pressure), difficulties with unexpected touch, or discomfort with certain types of physical contact. These sensitivities may impact greetings (handshakes, hugs), intimate relationships, or medical examinations, and may have significant social implications.

Temperature sensitivity might include heightened awareness of or discomfort with temperature variations that others might not notice, affecting environmental preferences and clothing choices. Some individuals may experience significant distress when too hot or too cold, beyond what would be expected based on the objective temperature.

Tactile assessment should also explore **potential hyposensitivity to touch or pain**, which might manifest as reduced awareness of injuries, temperature extremes, or uncomfortable physical positions. This reduced sensitivity can sometimes create safety risks if injuries go unnoticed or if the individual doesn't shift position when circulation is compromised.

Other sensory domains also warrant careful assessment, as they may significantly impact daily functioning:

Olfactory (smell) processing differences might include heightened awareness of and distress in response to odours that others might not notice, such as perfumes, cleaning products, or food smells. These sensitivities can affect where an individual can comfortably work, shop, or socialize, and may lead to significant limitations in community participation.

Gustatory (taste) sensitivities often interact with texture sensitivities to create food selectivity based on sensory properties rather than taste preferences alone. Assessment should explore whether food choices are limited based on sensory qualities such as texture, temperature, or flavour intensity, and whether this creates nutritional concerns or social limitations around shared meals.

Proprioceptive processing involves awareness of body position and movement. Differences in this system may manifest as unusual postures, difficulty grading movement force, clumsiness, or seeking deep pressure input. Some individuals may appear awkward in their movements or struggle with tasks requiring precise motor control.

Vestibular processing relates to balance and spatial orientation. Differences in this system might include unusual responses to movement, such as avoidance of certain movements (swings, elevators) or seeking intense vestibular input (spinning, rocking). Some individuals may experience significant distress with certain types of movement or positions.

Interoception refers to the perception of internal bodily sensations such as hunger, thirst, pain, or need for the toilet. Many adults with autism report reduced awareness of these internal signals, which can lead to difficulty with self-regulation of basic needs. Assessment should explore whether the individual has difficulty recognizing when they are hungry, thirsty, in pain, or need to use the bathroom, as these differences can have significant health implications.

Sensory processing differences often create cascading effects across multiple areas of functioning:

Emotional regulation may be significantly impacted by sensory input, with sensory overload often triggering anxiety, irritability, shutdown, or meltdown responses. Many adults with autism identify specific sensory triggers for emotional distress and may develop elaborate avoidance strategies to prevent exposure to these triggers.

Social participation can be limited by sensory sensitivities, as common social venues like restaurants, pubs, parties, or shopping centres may present overwhelming sensory environments. This can lead to social isolation that reflects sensory avoidance rather than lack of social interest.

Occupational functioning may be affected by sensory sensitivities to office environments, with fluorescent lighting, background conversations, ventilation system noises, or strong smells creating barriers to work performance. Appropriate accommodations for sensory needs can significantly improve occupational outcomes.

Daily living activities such as shopping, using public transportation, or attending healthcare appointments may be complicated by sensory challenges in these environments. Understanding these barriers is essential for developing effective support strategies.

Assessment of sensory processing should employ multiple methods to develop a comprehensive understanding of the individual's sensory profile:

Clinical interview should explore sensory experiences across all domains, identifying specific sensitivities, their intensity, contexts where they occur, and impact on daily functioning. Open-ended questions followed by specific probes about each sensory domain can elicit detailed information about sensory experiences that the individual may not have previously identified as relevant to their diagnosis.

Standardized measures such as the **Sensory Profile** (Adult version) provide a structured approach to assessing sensory processing patterns across multiple domains. This self-report questionnaire yields scores across sensory domains and processing patterns (seeking, avoiding, sensitivity, registration) that can be compared to normative data. Other measures such as the **Sensory Processing Quotient (SPQ)** may also provide valuable structured assessment of sensory features.

Observational assessment during the evaluation may reveal sensory behaviours such as covering ears in response to sounds, squinting under fluorescent lights, adjusting clothing repeatedly, or seeking certain sensory inputs through movement or touch. While some sensory responses may be deliberately masked during professional interactions, careful observation can still provide valuable information.

Environmental assessment, when possible, can provide insights into adaptations the individual has made to accommodate sensory needs. Home environments often reveal sensory preferences through lighting choices, sound management strategies, texture selections, or organization systems designed to create sensory comfort.

The assessment of sensory processing should ultimately aim to understand not only the pattern of sensitivities but also their impact on daily functioning and well-being. This comprehensive understanding can inform recommendations for environmental adaptations, coping strategies, and supports that respect the individual's sensory needs while addressing aspects that limit participation or cause distress. Effective sensory assessment and support can significantly improve quality of life for adults with autism, often representing one of the most immediately beneficial outcomes of the diagnostic process.

CHAPTER 16

Special Considerations in Adult Assessment

Assessing autism in adults presents unique challenges that differ significantly from childhood assessment. Several special considerations must be addressed to ensure accurate diagnosis and appropriate support planning for adults, particularly those without intellectual disabilities who may have developed sophisticated strategies to navigate social demands. Understanding these considerations is essential for clinicians working with adult populations, as they fundamentally shape the assessment approach and interpretation of findings.

Masking and camouflaging represent perhaps the most significant challenge in adult autism assessment, particularly for individuals with average or above-average cognitive abilities. These terms refer to the conscious or unconscious strategies used to hide or compensate for autism features in social situations. Masking involves the deliberate suppression of behaviours that might appear unusual (such as repetitive movements), while camouflaging involves the active performance of neurotypical-appearing social behaviours (such as making eye contact or using social phrases). Together, these strategies can create a presentation that obscures the underlying autism features, particularly in structured, time-limited assessment contexts.

Several dimensions of masking and camouflaging warrant careful consideration during assessment:

Deliberate compensation for social difficulties is common among adults with autism, particularly those who have received feedback throughout life about their social differences. These compensatory strategies might include rehearsing conversations in advance, memorizing appropriate phrases for specific social situations, deliberately monitoring facial expression and eye contact, or studying others' behaviour to determine appropriate responses. While these strategies may be effective in certain contexts, they typically require considerable cognitive effort and may break down in novel situations, during stress or fatigue, or in complex social interactions.

During assessment, these compensatory strategies may be identified through several approaches:

- noting inconsistencies in social performance across different contexts or topics
- observing signs of cognitive effort or fatigue during social interaction
- directly asking about strategies used to navigate social situations
- gathering collateral information about social functioning in less structured or more demanding contexts.

The artificial nature of the assessment setting, where social demands are relatively predictable and time-limited, may particularly facilitate effective compensation that might not be sustainable in real-world contexts.

Learned scripts and social routines represent a specific type of compensation where individuals develop standard responses or behaviours for common social situations. These might include greeting scripts, conversation starters, or pre-planned responses to typical questions. While these scripts may appear appropriate in isolation, they often lack the flexibility and spontaneity characteristic of neurotypical social interaction. During assessment, scripted responses may be identified by their somewhat formulaic nature, limited adaptation to the specific context, or breakdown when the interaction moves in unexpected directions.

"Social exhaustion" and burnout commonly result from the sustained effort required for masking and camouflaging. Many adults with autism report that while they can maintain neurotypical-appearing behaviour for certain periods, doing so is mentally exhausting and may lead to a need for solitary recovery time afterward. Some describe a pattern of "paying" for social engagement with periods of withdrawal or shutdown, or experiencing gradually declining social performance over the course of a day or week of high social demands. Assessment should explore not only whether the individual can perform socially but also the subjective experience and aftermath of that performance.

The assessment approach must be adapted to identify autism features that may be masked in formal settings. Strategies might include:

1. Extended assessment over multiple sessions, allowing observation of social performance as cognitive resources for compensation become depleted
2. Creating varied social contexts within the assessment, including both structured and unstructured interactions
3. Introducing unexpected elements that require spontaneous adaptation rather than rehearsed responses

4. Gathering detailed information about functioning across different environments and relationship contexts
5. Exploring the subjective experience of social interaction, including internal processes that may not be externally observable

Masking and camouflaging are particularly prevalent in certain populations, creating additional diagnostic challenges. Higher cognitive abilities generally facilitate more sophisticated compensation strategies, as intellectual strengths can be deployed to analyse and mimic social behaviour that does not come intuitively. This may contribute to the later diagnosis of individuals without intellectual disabilities, as their autism features may be less apparent in structured settings like school or healthcare appointments.

A higher prevalence of camouflaging has been consistently identified in females with autism, contributing to significant gender disparities in diagnosis rates. Research suggests that autistic females are more likely to study and imitate social behaviour, maintain a "social facade" in public while experiencing exhaustion afterward, and develop special interests that appear more socially acceptable. These gender-based camouflaging differences appear to reflect both biological factors and socialization pressures, as girls typically experience stronger expectations for social conformity and may receive earlier and more intensive feedback about social differences. The assessment of females should specifically address these camouflaging patterns, with recognition that standard instruments may be less sensitive to female presentations.

Late identification factors extend beyond masking to include various circumstances that may delay autism recognition until adulthood. Understanding these factors helps clinicians recognize how autism may have been overlooked despite being present throughout development.

High intelligence compensating for difficulties represents a common pathway to late diagnosis. Cognitive strengths may allow individuals to develop logical approaches to social interaction, excel in structured educational environments despite social challenges, or find niches where their cognitive abilities are valued and social differences are less important. Some adults with autism describe "solving" social interaction intellectually rather than processing it intuitively, using pattern recognition and logical analysis to navigate social demands that others process automatically. These compensations may be effective enough to prevent identification in childhood but still leave the individual feeling fundamentally different and experiencing significant effort and exhaustion from social demands.

Supportive environments masking challenges is another important consideration. Some individuals grow up in family, educational, or community contexts where their differences are accommodated without being labelled as clinical concerns. This might include families with similar cognitive styles (sometimes reflecting the broader autism phenotype in parents or siblings), educational settings that emphasize individual learning rather than social conformity, or communities that value the individual's specific strengths. While these accommodating environments can support healthy development, they may also delay identification of autism until the individual encounters fewer accommodating contexts in adulthood, such as higher education, employment, or romantic relationships where social expectations become more complex and less explicit.

Misdiagnosis and Diagnostic Overshadowing in Adult Autism

Misdiagnosis with other conditions commonly precedes adult autism diagnosis. Many adults report previous diagnoses of anxiety disorders, depression, personality disorders, psychotic disorders, or attention deficit hyperactivity disorder. While these conditions may genuinely co-occur with autism, in some cases they represent misinterpretations of autism features or secondary consequences of unrecognized autism. For example, social anxiety may be diagnosed when the underlying issue is social communication difficulty, or depression may be identified without recognition that it stems from chronic social challenges and sensory overload. Assessment should carefully explore previous mental health diagnoses, their response to typical treatments, and whether they might be better explained as aspects of autism or its consequences.

Exploring developmental history presents particular challenges in adult assessment but remains essential for diagnostic decision-making. Several approaches can enhance the quality of retrospective developmental information:

Retrospective recognition of traits involves helping the individual and informants identify patterns across development that may not have been previously recognized as autism-related. Specific, behavioural questions about childhood experiences often elicit more reliable information than general questions about autism features. For example, asking "*Did you have specific collections or interests that you spent a lot of time organizing or learning about?*" may be more effective than "*Did you have restricted interests as a child?*"

School reports and historical records can provide contemporaneous documentation of behaviours that may reflect unrecognized autism. Comments about social difficulties, rigid adherence to rules, unusual language patterns, specific intense interests, or sensory sensitivities may appear in these records without autism being considered at the time. These historical documents are particularly valuable as they are not subject to retrospective recall bias.

Patterns across different life stages should be explored to identify consistent traits despite changing manifestations. Autism features often present differently across development as the social environment changes and the individual develops coping strategies. For example, a young child's spinning or hand-flapping might evolve into an adult's leg bouncing or pen-clicking; a child's detailed dinosaur knowledge might transform into an adult's expertise in computer programming; or a child's social confusion might develop into an adult's social anxiety and avoidance. Identifying these developmental continuities can strengthen diagnostic confidence when current presentation is ambiguous.

The assessment of adults must consider how autism features may manifest differently across the lifespan, with recognition that adult presentation often differs from the childhood manifestations on which diagnostic criteria were primarily developed. Adults may have developed strategies to manage restricted and repetitive behaviours in public, found environments that accommodate their sensory needs, or created social scripts that work in predictable interactions. These adaptations don't negate the underlying autism but do require more sophisticated assessment approaches to identify.

Thoughtful adult assessment recognizes both the challenges of retrospective evaluation and the unique insights that adults can provide into their own developmental history and current internal experience. By combining skilled clinical interviewing, appropriate standardized measures, collateral information when available, and sensitivity to adult-specific manifestations of autism, clinicians can overcome the challenges of adult assessment to provide accurate diagnosis and meaningful support recommendations/camouflaging:

- Deliberate compensation for social difficulties
- Learned scripts and social routines
- "Social exhaustion" and burnout
- Higher prevalence in females and those with higher cognitive abilities
- Late identification factors:
  - High intelligence compensating for difficulties
  - Supportive environments masking challenges
  - Misdiagnosis with other conditions
- Exploring developmental history:
  - Retrospective recognition of traits
  - School reports and historical records
  - Patterns across different life stages

CHAPTER 17

Gender Differences in ASD Presentation

Understanding gender differences in autism presentation is essential for accurate diagnosis and appropriate support planning, particularly given the significant gender disparity in autism diagnosis rates. Historically, autism has been diagnosed more frequently in males, with ratios reported between 4:1 and 5:1 in many studies. However, growing evidence suggests that this disparity reflects diagnostic bias rather than true prevalence differences, with current research indicating that the actual male-to-female ratio may be closer to 3:2 or even 1:1 when accounting for underdiagnosis in females. This underdiagnosis stems from several factors, including gender-based variations in autism presentation, limitations in diagnostic tools developed primarily with male samples, and societal expectations that may mask or reinterpret autism features in females.

The concept of a distinct female autism phenotype has gained significant empirical support in recent years. This female presentation is not categorically different from male autism but represents a pattern of qualitative differences in how core autism features manifest. Understanding these gender-based variations is crucial for reducing diagnostic disparities and ensuring that females with autism receive appropriate identification and support.

More sophisticated social camouflaging represents one of the most significant gender differences in autism presentation. While both males and females with autism may develop compensatory strategies to navigate social demands, research consistently indicates that females employ these strategies more extensively and effectively. This enhanced camouflaging likely reflects both biological factors and strong socialization pressures, as females typically experience greater expectations for social conformity from an early age. The social camouflaging observed in females with autism often includes:

1. Careful observation and mimicry of socially successful peers, creating a "social toolkit" of behaviours and responses that can be deployed in various situations
2. Maintenance of a neurotypical-appearing social facade in public settings, often followed by exhaustion and need for recovery in private

3. Development of scripts and rehearsed responses for common social situations
4. Heightened awareness of and anxiety about social expectations and potential judgment
5. "Eclipsing" their own interests or preferences to align with peer groups

These camouflaging strategies may be so effective that autism features become apparent only in situations of high stress, novel social demands, or transitions where established compensation strategies are insufficient. Many females receive diagnosis only after such situations expose underlying difficulties that had previously been successfully masked.

The presentation of special interests may also differ by gender in ways that reduce identification of autism in females. While the intensity and focus of interests may be similar across genders, the content and social expression of these interests often follows gender-typical patterns that may appear less unusual to observers. Females with autism may develop intense interests in areas that seem more socially acceptable for their gender, such as animals, literature, psychology, arts, or certain celebrities or fictional characters. These interests might be mistaken for typical hobbies rather than recognized as having the intensity, focus, and systematic quality characteristic of autistic special interests.

Additionally, females may be more likely to share their interests in socially acceptable ways, finding peers with similar interests or modulating their discussion of interests based on social context. This social incorporation of special interests makes them less obvious as diagnostic indicators compared to the more socially isolated pursuit of interests often observed in males with autism. The assessment challenge lies in recognizing when apparently typical interests are pursued with unusual intensity, systematic focus, or collection of detailed information that distinguishes them from neurotypical hobbies.

The manifestation of social difficulties often differs qualitatively between males and females with autism. Males may present with more obvious social awkwardness, reduced social motivation, or clear difficulty understanding social rules. In contrast, females more commonly present with:

1. "Collecting" social behaviours through observation and systematic analysis rather than intuitive understanding
2. High social motivation despite significant social anxiety
3. Difficulty maintaining rather than initiating relationships
4. Vulnerability to social manipulation due to misreading intentions

5. Social exhaustion from the cognitive demands of managing social interactions
6. Relationship difficulties that become apparent primarily in complex or intimate relationships

These subtle social differences may not be immediately apparent in brief clinical encounters or structured settings but emerge in the detailed developmental history and reports of functioning across different social contexts. Many females with autism describe a sense of "social confusion" rather than disinterest, with strong desires for connection undermined by difficulty understanding the unwritten rules of social interaction.

The context-specific manifestation of social difficulties represents another important gender difference. Females with autism often show their most significant social challenges in specific contexts, while functioning adequately or even exceptionally in others. This variability may lead to dismissal of concerns when clinicians observe competent social performance in the assessment setting. Common patterns include:

1. Adequate functioning in one-to-one structured interactions (such as clinical assessment) but significant difficulties in group settings
2. Successful management of brief, scripted social exchanges but struggles with extended or open-ended social demands
3. Appropriate social behaviour in professional or educational contexts but exhaustion and withdrawal in personal settings
4. Successful navigation of childhood social demands but increasing difficulties as adolescent and adult social expectations become more complex and implicit

This context-dependent presentation necessitates gathering information about functioning across multiple environments rather than relying solely on observations in the assessment setting.

Assessment challenges created by gender differences require specific adaptations to standard diagnostic approaches. Traditional instruments developed and validated primarily with male samples may lack sensitivity to female manifestations of autism, contributing to underdiagnosis. The assessment of females should include:

1. Enhanced focus on camouflaging and compensation strategies, with explicit questioning about the cognitive effort required for social interaction, experiences of social exhaustion, and "passing as normal"

2. Exploration of how special interests manifest, looking beyond the content to examine the intensity, systematic approach, and immersive quality
3. Detailed examination of friendship patterns and relationship experiences rather than simply noting their presence or absence
4. Assessment of social understanding rather than just social behaviour, as performance may mask underlying difficulties
5. Exploration of sensory sensitivities and their management, which may be more prominent than obvious social or behavioural differences
6. Consideration of internalizing symptoms such as anxiety and depression, which may be secondary consequences of unrecognized autism

The lower sensitivity of current diagnostic criteria to female presentations remains a significant challenge. Diagnostic criteria were developed based primarily on male presentations, potentially missing the more subtle or qualitatively different manifestations in females. Clinicians should maintain awareness of this limitation and consider how core autism features might present differently while still reflecting the same underlying neurodevelopmental differences.

The higher threshold for clinical identification of females with autism operates at multiple levels. Parents and teachers may be less likely to raise concerns about girls with subtle social differences, attributing challenges instead to shyness, anxiety, or personality. Healthcare providers may not consider autism in females presenting with anxiety, eating disorders, or mood issues that might actually be secondary to underlying autism. Even when autism is considered, the presentation may not match clinicians' expectations based on more typical male presentations.

Assessment adaptations for females should include modifications to standard approaches to enhance sensitivity to female presentations:

1. Extended assessment over multiple sessions and contexts to observe social functioning when compensation strategies may be depleted
2. Careful probing for camouflaging strategies and their costs, including direct questions about the experience of "pretending to be normal" or "putting on a social mask"
3. Exploring friendship patterns in detail, including quality and reciprocity rather than just presence of relationships
4. Examining how special interests manifest and whether they follow gender-typical content areas while still showing unusual intensity or systematic focus

5. Gathering detailed developmental history with specific attention to subtle indicators that might have been overlooked
6. Using supplementary assessment tools developed with greater sensitivity to female presentations

The assessment process should also consider whether standard cut-off scores on diagnostic instruments are appropriate for females, as research suggests that lower thresholds may be needed to account for the more subtle presentation. Clinical judgment informed by understanding of gender differences becomes particularly important when standardized measures yield borderline or inconclusive results.

Gender-informed assessment is not about applying different diagnostic standards but rather ensuring that the same underlying neurodevelopmental condition is recognized across its varied manifestations. By understanding and actively assessing for gender-based variations in autism presentation, clinicians can help address the significant diagnostic disparities that have historically limited identification and support for females with autism. This more nuanced approach benefits all individuals with autism by expanding recognition beyond stereotypical presentations to encompass the true diversity of the autism spectrum.

CHAPTER 18

Cognitive Profile Assessment

Cognitive assessment provides valuable information that enhances understanding of an individual's strengths, challenges, and support needs within the context of autism assessment. While not mandatory for diagnosis, cognitive profiling offers insights into information processing, learning styles, and potential compensatory strategies that can inform both diagnostic decisions and post-diagnostic recommendations. The cognitive profiles associated with autism are diverse, reflecting the heterogeneity of the condition, but certain patterns occur with increased frequency and may provide supporting evidence for diagnosis when present.

Intelligence testing represents a common component of comprehensive autism assessment, with the **Wechsler Adult Intelligence Scale, Fourth Edition (WAIS-IV)** being the most widely used measure in UK clinical practice. This standardized assessment provides measures of verbal comprehension, perceptual reasoning, working memory, and processing speed, yielding both domain-specific and overall intelligence scores. Several aspects of **WAIS-IV** performance may be particularly informative in autism assessment:

Verbal versus performance discrepancies have historically been associated with autism, though the pattern and direction of these discrepancies vary considerably across individuals. Some adults with autism demonstrate significantly stronger perceptual reasoning than verbal comprehension, reflecting strengths in visual-spatial processing and logical reasoning paired with challenges in verbal concept formation and social language. Others show the opposite pattern, with strong verbal skills masking significant difficulties with perceptual integration or practical problem-solving. Still others show relatively even profiles across domains. The presence of significant discrepancies between verbal and performance abilities may suggest uneven development consistent with autism, though such discrepancies also occur in other conditions and are not diagnostic in isolation.

Peaks and troughs in subtest profile often provide more specific information than broad domain scores. Within the WAIS-IV, particular subtests may highlight cognitive patterns associated with autism. For example:

1. Block Design (a perceptual reasoning subtest involving constructing designs from blocks) often represents a relative strength in autism, reflecting enhanced local processing and attention to detail.
2. Matrix Reasoning (involving pattern completion and logical reasoning) may also be a relative strength, drawing on systematic thinking and pattern recognition.
3. Vocabulary and Similarities (verbal comprehension subtests) may show variable performance, with some individuals demonstrating extensive vocabulary but difficulty with abstract or social concepts.
4. Comprehension (measuring social reasoning and practical knowledge) frequently represents a relative weakness, reflecting challenges with social understanding and implicit knowledge.
5. Digit Span (a working memory measure) often shows better performance on straightforward repetition compared to mental manipulation of information, reflecting potential difficulties with cognitive flexibility.

The interpretation of intelligence testing results should consider several factors specific to autism assessment:

1. Performance may be affected by anxiety, sensory sensitivities in the testing environment, or difficulty understanding task demands due to language processing differences.
2. Standardized administration procedures may need adaptation to ensure valid results, such as providing additional clarification of instructions or allowing brief breaks to manage sensory overload or anxiety.
3. Intelligence scores should never be used as the sole basis for autism diagnostic decisions, as autism occurs across the full range of intellectual ability and IQ scores do not capture the qualitative differences in information processing that characterize autism.
4. Results should be interpreted within the context of the individual's educational and occupational history, as significant discrepancies between measured abilities and real-world achievement may provide insights into the impact of autism-related challenges.

Executive functioning assessment examines the cognitive processes involved in planning, organization, cognitive flexibility, response inhibition, and working memory. Difficulties in executive functioning are commonly associated with autism, though they are not universal or specific to the condition. Several aspects of executive functioning warrant specific assessment:

Planning and organization abilities affect how individuals approach complex tasks, manage time, and structure activities. Adults with autism often report difficulties with breaking down multi-step processes, estimating time requirements, or organizing materials and information. Assessment might include formal measures such as the Tower of London task (planning complex sequences) or the Rey Complex Figure Test (organization and planning in drawing), as well as structured clinical inquiry about real-world planning challenges.

Cognitive flexibility, sometimes called set-shifting, involves the ability to transition between different tasks, perspectives, or approaches. Difficulties with cognitive flexibility may manifest as perseveration (continuing with an approach despite feedback that it's not working), challenges with transitions between activities, or rigid application of rules across contexts where flexibility would be beneficial. The Wisconsin Card Sorting Test or the Trail Making Test (Part B) provides standardized assessment of set-shifting abilities, while clinical interview can explore real-world manifestations such as distress with changes in routine or difficulty adapting when plans change.

Response inhibition involves controlling impulses and suppressing automatic responses when inappropriate. Some adults with autism demonstrate challenges with inhibitory control, which may manifest as interrupting others in conversation, difficulty waiting their turn, or impulsively sharing thoughts without considering social appropriateness. The Stroop Test or Continuous Performance Tests can provide standardized measures of inhibitory control.

Working memory refers to the system for temporarily holding and manipulating information. Difficulties with working memory may affect conversation (forgetting earlier points while formulating a response), complex task completion (losing track of steps in a sequence), or following multi-step instructions. Working memory can be assessed through subtests of the WAIS-IV (Digit Span, Letter-Number Sequencing) or specialized measures like the N-back task.

When assessing executive functioning, it's important to recognize that performance in structured assessment settings may not fully capture real-world challenges. Many adults with autism demonstrate adequate performance on laboratory measures of executive functioning but struggle significantly with the application of these skills in complex, dynamic real-world settings. Complementing standardized assessment with detailed discussion of daily functioning can provide a more comprehensive understanding of executive functioning strengths and challenges.

Central Coherence and Cognitive Style in Autism

Central coherence refers to the cognitive tendency to process information in context for global meaning, often at the expense of attention to detail. The theory of weak central coherence in autism suggests a processing bias toward local details rather than global integration. This cognitive style is not necessarily a deficit but represents a different way of processing information that can be advantageous in some contexts while creating challenges in others.

Assessment of central coherence might include:

1. The Embedded Figures Test, which measures the ability to identify simple shapes within complex designs, with enhanced performance often observed in autism
2. The Navon task, using large letters composed of smaller letters to assess preference for local versus global processing
3. The Homograph Reading Task, examining the use of context to determine the appropriate pronunciation of ambiguous words
4. The Block Design subtest from the WAIS-IV, particularly examining whether designs are approached as integrated wholes or component parts

Local versus global processing tendencies may also be observed qualitatively during other assessment activities, such as storytelling (focus on details versus central themes), description of social situations (attention to specific behaviours versus overall social meaning), or conversation (focus on specific words or phrases versus overall communicative intent).

Theory of mind assessment examines the understanding of others' mental states, including their beliefs, intentions, desires, and emotions. Differences in theory of mind processing have been consistently associated with autism, though the nature and extent of these differences vary considerably across individuals and development. Assessment might include:

1. Advanced theory of mind tasks such as the Strange Stories Test, which presents vignettes requiring understanding of non-literal language, deception, or complex social motivations
2. The Faux Pas Recognition Test, examining the ability to identify and explain social missteps
3. The Reading the Mind in the Eyes Test, assessing emotion recognition from subtle facial cues
4. Video-based tasks presenting social scenarios and assessing understanding of characters' intentions and emotions

Theory of mind assessment should consider both explicit reasoning (the ability to explain others' mental states when specifically prompted) and implicit, real-time social understanding (the automatic integration of mental state information during ongoing social interaction). Many adults with autism develop explicit theory of mind skills through cognitive strategies and learning but continue to experience challenges with the rapid, automatic social processing required in dynamic interactions.

Language pragmatics assessment examines the social use of language beyond vocabulary and grammar, including conversational turn-taking, topic maintenance, narrative coherence, understanding of non-literal language, and adaptation of communication to different social contexts. Pragmatic language differences are central to the social communication challenges in autism and warrant specific assessment:

1. Standardized measures such as the Test of Pragmatic Language or the Communication Checklist - Adult Version can provide structured assessment of pragmatic skills
2. Analysis of narrative samples, examining story structure, reference clarity, and integration of elements
3. Assessment of figurative language comprehension, including idioms, metaphors, humour, and sarcasm
4. Observation of conversational skills across different topics and contexts

Pragmatic language assessment is particularly relevant for adults with strong structural language abilities (vocabulary and grammar), where social communication difficulties may primarily reflect challenges with the pragmatic aspects of language rather than basic language skills.

The cognitive assessment approach should be tailored to the individual's presentation, referral questions, and assessment context. Comprehensive cognitive assessment is not mandatory for autism diagnosis, and the selection of specific measures should be guided by clinical judgment regarding which aspects of cognition will provide the most relevant information for that individual. Several factors influence this decision:

1. Time constraints and service resources may limit the feasibility of comprehensive cognitive assessment, necessitating prioritization of the most informative measures
2. Previous cognitive assessments may already provide relevant information, reducing the need for repeat testing
3. The individual's presenting concerns and functional challenges should guide the focus of cognitive assessment

4. The complexity of the diagnostic picture may warrant more or less extensive cognitive assessment to clarify the presentation

When cognitive assessment is included, it should be approached not as a way to diagnose autism but as a method for developing a more nuanced understanding of the individual's information processing style, learning approach, and support needs. The integration of cognitive findings with other assessment information enhances the development of personalized support recommendations that leverage cognitive strengths while addressing areas of challenge.

CHAPTER 19

Differential Diagnosis - Overview

Differential diagnosis—the process of distinguishing autism from other conditions with overlapping features—represents a critical component of comprehensive assessment. Accurate differential diagnosis ensures that individuals receive appropriate diagnoses and interventions while avoiding misattribution of symptoms that might better be explained by other conditions. This process is particularly challenging in adult assessment due to the complex presentations that may include multiple co-occurring conditions, long-standing compensatory strategies, and the impact of previous diagnoses and treatments on current functioning.

Several core differential considerations must be systematically evaluated during autism assessment. These conditions share features with autism but differ in important ways that affect diagnostic decision-making and intervention planning:

Social anxiety disorder (SAD) & Its distinctions

Social anxiety disorder (SAD) frequently presents with social avoidance, discomfort in social situations, and difficulty with social interaction that may superficially resemble autism. However, important distinctions include:

1. **The nature of social difficulties**: In SAD, social skills and understanding are typically intact, but anxiety interferes with their execution. In autism, fundamental differences in social cognition and communication exist independent of anxiety.
2. **Developmental history**: SAD often emerges in late childhood or adolescence, while autism features are present from early development, though they may become more apparent as social demands increase.
3. **Response to social success**: Individuals with SAD typically experience reduced anxiety following successful social interactions, while those with autism may continue to find social interaction effortful or confusing despite apparent success.

4. **Breadth of symptoms**: SAD primarily affects social functioning, without the restricted interests, repetitive behaviours, or sensory sensitivities characteristic of autism.

It's important to note that SAD frequently co-occurs with autism, with some studies suggesting that up to 50% of adults with autism experience clinically significant social anxiety. This co-occurrence can complicate differential diagnosis and requires careful assessment of the temporal relationship between social anxiety and social communication differences, as well as the presence of autism features beyond the social domain.

Obsessive-compulsive disorder (OCD)

Obsessive-compulsive disorder (OCD) shares features with the restricted and repetitive behaviour domain of autism, including ritualized behaviours, insistence on sameness, and intense preoccupations. Differentiating factors include:

1. **Ego-dystonic versus ego-syntonic nature**: In OCD, rituals and compulsions are typically experienced as unwanted and distressing, performed to neutralize anxiety rather than for inherent enjoyment. In autism, repetitive behaviours and routines are often experienced as pleasurable, calming, or simply preferred.
2. **Content of preoccupations**: OCD obsessions typically focus on harm, contamination, symmetry, or taboo thoughts, while autism special interests usually involve intense fascination with specific topics or systems.
3. **Social and communication development**: OCD does not typically involve the persistent social communication differences characteristic of autism.
4. **Response to treatment**: OCD typically responds to specific cognitive-behavioural approaches (exposure and response prevention) and serotonergic medications, while these interventions do not affect core autism features.

Like SAD, OCD frequently co-occurs with autism, requiring careful assessment of whether repetitive behaviours and preoccupations reflect OCD, autism, or both conditions simultaneously.

Personality disorders, particularly schizoid, schizotypal, and avoidant types, share some features with autism and may be misdiagnosed in adults with unrecognized autism. Key distinctions include:

Schizoid personality disorder involves limited interest in social relationships and restricted emotional expression, potentially resembling the social differences in autism. However, individuals with schizoid personality disorder typically do not desire social relationships and are comfortable with their solitude, while many individuals with autism desire connection but struggle with social understanding and execution. Additionally, schizoid personality disorder does not involve the restricted interests, repetitive behaviours, or sensory sensitivities seen in autism.

Schizotypal personality disorder includes odd thinking, unusual perceptual experiences, and social difficulties that might be confused with autism features. The key distinctions involve the nature of unusual thinking (magical or paranoid ideation in schizotypal personality disorder versus logical but rigid thinking in autism) and the quality of social difficulties (social anxiety and paranoia in schizotypal personality disorder versus fundamental social communication differences in autism).

Avoidant personality disorder involves social avoidance driven by fear of criticism or rejection, which might be confused with the social withdrawal seen in some individuals with autism. The distinguishing features include the motivation for social avoidance (fear of negative evaluation in avoidant personality disorder versus social confusion or overwhelm in autism) and the presence of autism features beyond the social domain.

For all personality disorders, a crucial differentiating factor is developmental history. Personality disorders, by definition, involve enduring patterns of inner experience and behavior that deviate from cultural norms, with onset in adolescence or early adulthood. Autism, as a neurodevelopmental condition, is present from early childhood, though recognition may be delayed. Careful developmental assessment can help distinguish between these conditions.

Attention deficit hyperactivity disorder (ADHD) shares several features with autism, including social difficulties, sensory sensitivities, and executive functioning challenges. The high rate of co-occurrence between these conditions (30-80% of adults with autism have ADHD symptoms) further complicates differential diagnosis. Key distinctions include:

1. **Primary attention deficits versus attention to preferred interests**: In ADHD, attention difficulties are generally pervasive, though they may improve with high interest or novelty. In autism, attention may be exceptionally focused on preferred interests while being significantly reduced for non-preferred activities.
2. **Impulsivity versus social disinhibition**: In ADHD, impulsivity reflects difficulty suppressing automatic responses across contexts. In autism, apparent impulsivity in social situations may reflect misunderstanding of social norms rather than general inhibitory control deficits.

3. **Hyperactivity versus repetitive movements**: The hyperactivity of ADHD typically involves general restlessness and difficulty remaining still, while repetitive movements in autism are often more specific and patterned, serving sensory or regulatory functions.
4. **Social difficulties**: In ADHD, social challenges often relate to impulsivity, inattention to social cues, or disruptive behaviour. In autism, social difficulties reflect fundamental differences in social cognition and communication.

The frequent co-occurrence of autism and ADHD necessitates careful assessment of both conditions, with recognition that an individual may meet criteria for both diagnoses. UK clinical practice, following ICD-11 guidance, now recognizes these conditions can co-occur, representing an important shift from previous diagnostic approaches that considered them mutually exclusive.

Language disorders with social impact may present with communication difficulties that resemble autism. Conditions such as developmental language disorder with pragmatic features or semantic-pragmatic language disorder involve challenges with the social use of language that can appear similar to the social communication differences in autism. Distinguishing features include:

1. **Presence of restricted and repetitive behaviours**: Language disorders do not typically involve the restricted interests, repetitive behaviours, or sensory sensitivities characteristic of autism.
2. **Non-verbal social communication**: Individuals with primary language disorders often compensate effectively with non-verbal communication (gesture, facial expression, etc.), while those with autism typically show differences across verbal and non-verbal social communication.
3. **Social motivation and understanding**: Those with language disorders typically demonstrate age-appropriate social interest and understanding despite expressive language limitations, while social cognition differences are central to autism.

Assessment tools such as the **Children's Communication Checklist-2** or the **Clinical Evaluation of Language Fundamentals (CELF-5)** can help differentiate language disorders from autism, though specialized speech and language therapy assessment may be necessary in complex cases.

Intellectual disability frequently co-occurs with autism (approximately 30% co-occurrence), but can also present with social and behavioural features that might be mistaken for autism in the absence of true social communication differences. Careful assessment must distinguish:

1. Social difficulties due to cognitive limitations versus qualitative differences in social understanding
2. Repetitive behaviours related to developmental level versus those characteristics of autism
3. Communication challenges proportionate to general cognitive functioning versus specific pragmatic language differences

Assessment of autism in the context of intellectual disability requires adaptation of standard approaches, with greater emphasis on observation, informant report, and developmental history, as self-report and some standardized measures may be less accessible or valid.

Psychotic disorders, particularly schizophrenia with negative symptoms (reduced emotional expression, social withdrawal) might be confused with autism, especially in first presentations. Important distinctions include:

1. **Developmental history**: Schizophrenia typically emerges in late adolescence or early adulthood, while autism features are present from early childhood.
2. **Presence of positive psychotic symptoms** (hallucinations, delusions) in schizophrenia but not autism
3. **Nature of thinking differences**: Logical but rigid thinking in autism versus disorganized or delusional thinking in schizophrenia
4. **Response to antipsychotic medication**: Effective for psychotic symptoms but not core autism features

Diagnostic hierarchy considerations should guide the overall approach to differential diagnosis. When multiple conditions may be present, clinicians must determine which represent primary versus secondary presentations. Several principles inform this hierarchy:

1. **Developmental primacy**: Conditions present from early development typically have formative effects on subsequent development and adaptation
2. **Causal relationships**: Some conditions may arise as consequences or complications of others
3. **Treatment implications**: Prioritizing conditions with specific, effective treatments may guide intervention planning
4. **Functional impact**: Conditions causing the most significant impairment may warrant primary clinical attention

The concept of diagnostic overshadowing is particularly relevant in autism assessment. This occurs when co-occurring conditions are misattributed to autism or when autism is overlooked due to more obvious psychiatric presentations. Careful attention to the specific features, developmental course, and response to previous interventions for each condition can help avoid diagnostic overshadowing in either direction.

UK diagnostic practice follows ICD-11 criteria and coding, which has evolved significantly in recent revisions. Key changes relevant to differential diagnosis include:

1. Reclassification of autism as "autism spectrum disorder" without the previous subtypes (e.g., Asperger's syndrome)
2. Recognition that autism can co-occur with other neurodevelopmental conditions including ADHD
3. Introduction of specifiers for intellectual functioning and functional language
4. Increased recognition of sensory processing differences as core features

These diagnostic framework changes support more nuanced differential diagnosis that recognizes the complex patterns of co-occurrence often seen in clinical practice. The differential diagnostic process should ultimately aim not simply to determine which single diagnosis best explains the presentation, but to develop a comprehensive formulation that accounts for the individual's unique pattern of strengths, challenges, and support needs across multiple domains of functioning.

CHAPTER 20

Differential Diagnosis - Social Communication Disorders

Social (Pragmatic) Communication Disorder (SCD) represents one of the most challenging differential diagnoses in autism assessment, as it shares the social communication difficulties characteristic of autism but without the restricted and repetitive behaviour patterns. Understanding the distinctions between these conditions is essential for accurate diagnosis and appropriate intervention planning, particularly since their optimal supports may differ significantly.

Social (Pragmatic) Communication Disorder emerged as a distinct diagnostic category in DSM-5 and subsequently in ICD-11, where it is classified as "developmental language disorder with impairment mainly affecting pragmatic language." This diagnostic category was developed partly in response to concerns about individuals who demonstrated significant social communication challenges but did not meet full criteria for autism spectrum disorder, particularly following the removal of Asperger's syndrome as a separate diagnosis. The core features of SCD include:

1. Persistent difficulties with the social use of verbal and nonverbal communication, including:
    - Difficulty with communication appropriate to social context
    - Challenges with following rules of conversation and storytelling
    - Problems understanding non-literal language and implied meanings
    - Difficulty adjusting communication to match audience needs
2. These difficulties result in functional limitations in effective communication, social participation, academic achievement, or occupational performance
3. The onset of symptoms occurs in the early developmental period

4. The difficulties are not better explained by autism spectrum disorder, intellectual disability, global developmental delay, or another mental disorder

The crucial diagnostic distinction is that SCD does not include the restricted, repetitive patterns of behaviour, interests, or activities that are required for an autism diagnosis. In practice, this differentiation requires careful assessment of whether truly no restricted or repetitive behaviours are present, or whether they are simply less obvious or have been masked by developmental adaptations.

The development of this diagnostic category in DSM-5/ICD-11 reflected several clinical and research considerations:

1. Recognition that social communication difficulties exist on a continuum, with some individuals presenting with significant challenges that affect functioning but do not meet full autism criteria
2. Concern that the removal of Asperger's syndrome as a separate diagnosis might leave some individuals without access to appropriate diagnostic recognition and services
3. Growing understanding of the heterogeneity of pragmatic language difficulties and their relationship to both autism and language disorders
4. Need for specific intervention approaches targeting social communication that might differ from typical autism interventions

The validity and utility of SCD as a distinct diagnostic category remain subjects of ongoing research and clinical debate. Some researchers question whether it represents a truly distinct condition or simply reflects autism with less obvious restricted and repetitive behaviours. Others view it as a valuable diagnostic category that recognizes the significant functional impact of social communication difficulties even in the absence of other autism features. This debate highlights the importance of thorough assessment that examines not only current presentation but developmental history and functioning across contexts.

Several language disorders with social impact may present similarly to autism or SCD, requiring careful differential diagnosis:

1. Developmental language disorder with pragmatic features involves difficulties with the social use of language in the context of broader language development challenges. Unlike autism, these difficulties are primarily related to language development rather than broader social cognition differences. Assessment should examine whether social difficulties extend beyond language-based interaction and whether they persist in contexts with reduced language demands.

2. Semantic-pragmatic language disorder, a term more commonly used in UK clinical practice than in formal diagnostic systems, describes a pattern of language development characterized by fluent but unusual language, difficulty with language comprehension, and pragmatic language challenges. This presentation shares features with both autism and developmental language disorder, highlighting the complex overlaps between these conditions. Current diagnostic frameworks generally conceptualize semantic-pragmatic language disorder as either a subtype of developmental language disorder or a presentation of autism with prominent language features, rather than as a distinct condition.

Distinguishing features that help differentiate these language disorders from autism include:

- Developmental trajectory represents a key distinguishing factor. While both autism and language disorders are developmental conditions, their patterns of emergence and progression often differ. Language disorders typically present with early delays or differences in language acquisition as the primary concern, with social difficulties becoming more apparent as language demands increase. In contrast, autism often involves early differences in social engagement, joint attention, and play alongside communication development.
- Pattern of difficulties across contexts can provide important diagnostic information. Language disorders primarily affect functioning in contexts with high language demands, while autism typically impacts social functioning across contexts, including those with minimal language requirements. Careful assessment of functioning across different environments and relationship types can help identify whether social difficulties persist beyond language-based interactions.
- Response to language-focused interventions may also differentiate these conditions. Individuals with primary language disorders often show significant improvement in social functioning when provided with appropriate language supports and interventions. While individuals with autism also benefit from language intervention, their social differences typically require additional social cognition and interaction-focused approaches.

Assessment tools specific to language functioning can contribute valuable information to the differential diagnostic process. These include:

1. The **Clinical Evaluation of Language Fundamentals (CELF-5)** that provides comprehensive assessment of language skills across domains, including pragmatic language. The CELF-5 includes both direct

assessment tasks and observation scales, offering insights into both structural and social aspects of language.

2. The **Children's Communication Checklist-2 (CCC-2)**, despite its name, can be useful for young adults up to age 21. This informant-report measure specifically examines communication skills across domains including pragmatics, social interaction, and language structure. The profile of scores across scales can help differentiate between primarily structural language difficulties and the social communication patterns more characteristic of autism.
3. The **Test of Pragmatic Language-2 (TOPL-2)** directly assesses pragmatic language skills through scenarios requiring understanding of social communication rules. Performance on this measure can highlight specific areas of pragmatic difficulty and their relationship to overall language functioning.
4. The **La Trobe Communication Questionnaire** examines communication skills in everyday contexts, providing information about functional communication that may not be apparent in structured assessment settings.

When language disorders are suspected, referral for specialized speech and language therapy assessment is often warranted. Speech and language therapists bring specific expertise in distinguishing between different patterns of language development and can provide detailed assessment of pragmatic language functioning that enhances the diagnostic process.

Several clinical considerations are important when differentiating between autism, SCD, and language disorders:

1. These conditions exist on continua with complex overlaps rather than as discrete categories with clear boundaries. Some individuals may present with features that do not neatly fit a single diagnostic category, requiring careful formulation that captures their unique profile.
2. Co-occurrence is common, with many individuals meeting criteria for both autism and language disorders. In such cases, both diagnoses may be appropriate to ensure access to comprehensive intervention approaches.
3. Developmental changes may affect presentation over time, with some individuals showing shifts in their profile of strengths and challenges throughout development. A diagnosis that accurately reflected presentation in early childhood might need reconsideration in adulthood.
4. Cultural and linguistic diversity significantly impacts assessment of social communication, as pragmatic rules vary considerably across cultures and

languages. Assessment must consider the individual's cultural and linguistic background when determining whether communication patterns represent disorder or cultural difference.

5. Gender differences may affect presentation, with females sometimes showing stronger structural language skills that mask underlying pragmatic difficulties. This can contribute to underdiagnosis of both autism and social communication disorders in females.

The differential diagnosis process should ultimately focus not simply on determining which diagnostic label best applies, but on developing a nuanced understanding of the individual's communication profile that can inform personalized intervention approaches. This may include consideration of:

1. Specific patterns of pragmatic language strengths and challenges
2. Relationship between language skills and social functioning
3. Contexts where communication difficulties are most and least apparent
4. Impact of communication challenges on educational, occupational, and social outcomes
5. Previous response to communication-focused interventions

This comprehensive understanding, rather than diagnostic categorization alone, provides the foundation for effective support planning that addresses the individual's unique needs, whether they ultimately receive a diagnosis of autism, Social (Pragmatic) Communication Disorder, or a language disorder.

CHAPTER 21

Differential Diagnosis - Personality Disorders

Personality disorders, particularly those in Cluster A (schizoid, schizotypal) and Cluster C (avoidant), share several features with autism spectrum disorder that can create significant diagnostic challenges. The overlap between these conditions is particularly relevant in adult assessment, as personality disorders are, by definition, diagnosed in adulthood based on enduring patterns of inner experience and behaviour. Understanding the distinctions between autism and various personality disorders is essential for accurate diagnosis and appropriate intervention planning.

Schizoid Personality Disorder (SPD) presents with a pattern of detachment from social relationships and restricted emotional expression, features that may superficially resemble the social differences observed in autism. According to ICD-11, key characteristics of SPD include:

1. Emotional detachment and reduced capacity for emotional experience and expression
2. Limited capacity to experience pleasure (anhedonia)
3. Apparent indifference to praise, criticism, or others' feelings
4. Limited interest in sexual experiences with others
5. Preference for solitary activities and limited interest in social relationships
6. Limited introspection and self-awareness

The substantial overlap with autism features creates significant differential diagnostic challenges. However, several key distinctions can guide the assessment process:

Limited interest in relationships versus difficulty with social understanding represents perhaps the most crucial distinction. Individuals with SPD typically have little desire for close relationships and are content with their solitude. In contrast, many individuals with autism desire social connection but struggle with understanding social dynamics, reading social cues, or executing appropriate social behaviours. This distinction is not absolute—some individuals with autism may indeed have limited social motivation, while some with SPD may have a degree of social interest—but exploring the subjective experience of social disconnection often reveals meaningful differences.

During assessment, direct questioning about social motivation can be illuminating: "Do you wish you had more friends or closer relationships?" "Do you enjoy spending time with others when social interaction goes well?" "Do you feel lonely or do you prefer being alone?" Individuals with autism often express loneliness, confusion about why relationships are difficult, or desire for connection despite their challenges, while those with SPD typically report comfort with solitude and limited interest in increasing social engagement.

The absence of desire for relationships versus unsuccessful attempts represents another important distinction. Individuals with SPD generally do not attempt to form close relationships and may actively avoid them. In contrast, many individuals with autism make efforts to connect with others but struggle with the execution of social interaction or understanding unwritten social rules. Assessment should explore not only current social networks but also the history of relationship attempts, responses to social failure, and feelings about social isolation.

It's important to note that distinguishing between lack of social motivation and social avoidance due to repeated failure can be challenging. Some adults with autism develop secondary social avoidance after years of negative social experiences, potentially resembling the presentation of SPD. Careful developmental history is essential for understanding whether current social patterns reflect lifelong preference or adaptation to social challenges.

The quality of emotional expression also differs between these conditions. In SPD, restricted emotional expression stems from genuinely limited emotional experience—a reduced capacity for both positive and negative emotions. In autism, emotional experiences are often intense but may be expressed atypically or inconsistently. Many adults with autism report feeling emotions deeply but struggling to identify, regulate, or communicate their emotional states in conventional ways. Assessment should explore not only observed emotional expression but also subjective emotional experience, including intensity, awareness, and communication of emotions.

The presence of restricted and repetitive behaviours represents a defining feature of autism that is not characteristic of SPD. While individuals with SPD may have circumscribed interests, these typically lack the intensity, focused attention to detail, or systematic quality that characterizes autism special interests. Similarly, the sensory sensitivities, movement differences, and need for sameness common in autism are not features of SPD. Thorough assessment of the restricted and repetitive behaviour domain can provide crucial information for differential diagnosis.

Schizotypal Personality Disorder presents with unusual perceptions and beliefs, cognitive and perceptual distortions, eccentricities in behaviour and appearance, and social difficulties. According to ICD-11, key features include:

1. Odd beliefs, magical thinking, or paranoid ideas
2. Unusual perceptual experiences including bodily illusions
3. Odd thinking and speech (vague, metaphorical, over-elaborate)
4. Suspiciousness or paranoid ideas
5. Inappropriate or constricted affect
6. Eccentric behaviour or appearance
7. Limited close relationships and social anxiety

Several features overlap with autism, creating potential diagnostic confusion. However, important distinctions can guide differential diagnosis:

1. **Unusual perceptions versus sensory sensitivities** represent different types of sensory experiences. In schizotypal personality disorder, unusual perceptions often involve illusions, bodily distortions, or quasi-psychotic experiences like sensing a presence. In autism, sensory differences typically involve hypersensitivity or hyposensitivity to ordinary sensory input (lights, sounds, textures) rather than perceptual distortions. While both conditions involve atypical sensory experiences, the quality and nature of these experiences differ substantially.

Assessment should carefully explore the specific nature of sensory experiences: "Do ordinary sounds, lights, or textures bother you more than they seem to bother other people?" (common in autism) versus "Do you ever feel like your body is changing shape or size, or sense things that others can't see or hear?" (more characteristic of schizotypal personality disorder).

2. **Odd thinking versus special interests** reflects different cognitive patterns. The odd thinking in schizotypal personality disorder typically involves magical thinking, ideas of reference, or unusual beliefs that may approach but not reach delusional intensity. In contrast, the special interest's characteristic of autism involves intense focus on specific topics, often with logical but highly detailed thinking rather than magical or unusual beliefs. While both conditions may involve unusual conversations,

the content and quality differ—schizotypal speech often being vague, tangential, or metaphorical, while autistic speech about special interests is typically fact-focused, detailed, and logical (though sometimes pedantic).

Assessment should explore not only the topics of interest but the cognitive approach to these topics: "Do you notice connections between unrelated events that others don't see?" (more characteristic of schizotypal personality disorder) versus "Do you collect detailed information about specific topics that interest you?" (more characteristic of autism).

3. **Social disinhibition versus social communication differences** also distinguishes these conditions. The social difficulties in schizotypal personality disorder often involve suspiciousness, ideas of reference (believing neutral events relate to oneself), and social anxiety based on concerns about others' intentions. In autism, social difficulties typically stem from challenges with understanding social cues, pragmatic language differences, and difficulty with the reciprocal nature of social interaction. These different mechanisms lead to distinct patterns of social behaviour that careful assessment can differentiate.

Avoidant Personality Disorder involves a pattern of social inhibition, feelings of inadequacy, and hypersensitivity to negative evaluation. According to ICD-11, key features include:

1. Extensive pattern of avoidance of social situations and restraint in social situations due to fear of rejection or disapproval
2. Persistent and pervasive feelings of tension and apprehension
3. Belief that one is socially inept, personally unappealing, or inferior to others
4. Excessive preoccupation with being criticized or rejected in social situations
5. Unwillingness to become involved with people unless certain of being liked
6. Restricted lifestyle due to need for physical security
7. Avoidance of social or occupational activities involving significant interpersonal contact

The social avoidance characteristic of this condition may resemble the social difficulties seen in some presentations of autism, particularly in adults who have developed social anxiety after negative social experiences. However, several key distinctions guide differential diagnosis:

Fear of rejection versus lack of social understanding reflects different mechanisms underlying social difficulties. In avoidant personality disorder, social avoidance stems from fear of criticism, rejection, or negative evaluation, despite adequate social skills and understanding. In autism, social challenges primarily reflect differences in social cognition, pragmatic language, and nonverbal communication, though secondary social anxiety may develop over time.

Assessment should explore the subjective experience of social situations: "What makes social situations difficult for you?" "What are you concerned might happen in social situations?" "Have you always found social situations challenging, or did this develop at a particular time?" Individuals with avoidant personality disorder typically identify fear of judgment or rejection as primary concerns, while those with autism more often describe confusion about social expectations, difficulty processing social information in real time, or sensory aspects of social environments.

Desire for relationships with anxiety versus reduced social motivation or understanding represents another important distinction. Individuals with avoidant personality disorder typically desire close relationships but avoid them due to fear of rejection, while the social patterns in autism may reflect fundamental differences in social cognition or communication rather than primarily anxiety-driven avoidance. Assessment should explore whether the individual wishes for more social connection but feels afraid, or whether they struggle with understanding and executing the social behaviours necessary for relationship development.

Presence of restricted and repetitive behaviours, as with other personality disorders, provides a key distinguishing feature. The restricted and repetitive behaviours characteristic of autism—including special interests, sensory sensitivities, and need for sameness—are not features of avoidant personality disorder. Thorough assessment of this domain helps differentiate between these conditions and identify whether social avoidance exists in isolation or as part of a broader autism presentation.

Assessment approach considerations for differentiating autism from personality disorders include:

Developmental history provides crucial information, as autism is a neurodevelopmental condition present from early childhood, while personality disorders typically emerge in adolescence or early adulthood. Assessment should carefully explore early development, including:

1. Early social engagement, joint attention, and play patterns
2. Language development, including pragmatic aspects
3. Presence of restricted interests, repetitive behaviours, or sensory sensitivities in childhood

4. Patterns of peer relationships throughout development
5. Age of onset for social difficulties and their evolution over time

Consistent evidence of autism features from early development strongly supports an autism diagnosis, while patterns that emerge primarily in adolescence or adulthood may more likely reflect personality disorders (though early, subtle autism features are sometimes recognized only in retrospect).

Quality of social understanding versus avoidance distinguishes between fundamentally different social mechanisms. Assessment should examine not only whether the individual engages in social interaction but their understanding of social dynamics, ability to read social cues, and quality of social reciprocity when they do engage socially. Individuals with personality disorders typically demonstrate better social understanding than social performance would suggest, while those with autism often show consistent differences in social cognition even when motivated to engage socially.

Structured assessment tools may help differentiate these conditions. While no measures specifically target this differential diagnosis, autism-specific instruments like the **ADOS-2** and **ADI-R** assess features not characteristic of personality disorders, while personality measures like the Structured Clinical Interview for **DSM Personality Disorders (SCID-5-PD)** explore features specific to personality disorders. When used together, these complementary approaches can help distinguish between these conditions.

It's important to recognize that autism and personality disorders can co-occur, with some individuals meeting criteria for both conditions. In such cases, understanding the developmental sequence helps clarify whether personality patterns developed as adaptations to underlying autism or represent distinct co-occurring conditions. Either way, comprehensive formulation that addresses both neurodevelopmental and personality factors provides the foundation for effective intervention planning.

CHAPTER 22

Differential Diagnosis - ADHD

Attention Deficit Hyperactivity Disorder (ADHD) represents one of the most complex and challenging differential diagnoses in adult autism assessment. The substantial symptom overlap, frequent co-occurrence, and shared neurodevelopmental origins of these conditions create significant complexity in the diagnostic process. According to Rommelse et al. (2017), "Autism and ADHD show significant clinical, genetic and neurobiological overlap and can be considered as different manifestations of a common underlying disorder" (p.428).

The overlap between autism and ADHD is extensive and spans multiple domains of functioning. Both conditions involve neurodevelopmental differences that emerge early in development, persist throughout the lifespan, and affect functioning across contexts. The specific areas of overlap include:

Social communication difficulties appear in both conditions but stem from different underlying mechanisms. In ADHD, social challenges typically result from executive functioning difficulties that affect social attention, impulse control, and conversational regulation. Individuals with ADHD may interrupt conversations, miss social cues due to inattention, struggle with waiting their turn, or have difficulty sustaining focus during social interactions. These difficulties occur despite generally intact social cognition and understanding of social norms. In contrast, the social communication difficulties in autism reflect more fundamental differences in social cognition, pragmatic language understanding, and nonverbal communication processing (Nijmeijer et al., 2008).

The behavioural manifestations of these different underlying mechanisms can appear remarkably similar in clinical settings. Both individuals with ADHD and those with autism may demonstrate poor eye contact, difficulty with conversational turn-taking, problems maintaining friendships, and social awkwardness. This surface-level similarity necessitates careful assessment of the underlying reasons for these social behaviours rather than relying solely on their presence or absence.

Executive functioning challenges are prominent in both conditions but may show different patterns. ADHD is fundamentally a disorder of executive function, particularly affecting attention regulation, inhibitory control, and working memory. Executive functioning difficulties in autism, while common, are more variable across individuals and may particularly affect cognitive flexibility, planning, and generalization of skills across contexts (Demetriou et al., 2018).

The executive functioning profiles often overlap significantly, with both conditions associated with difficulties in organization, time management, task initiation, and completion of multi-step activities. However, subtle differences may be observed like individuals with ADHD typically show more consistent difficulties with sustained attention and impulse control across contexts, while those with autism may demonstrate excellent sustained attention for preferred activities alongside significant challenges with set-shifting and adapting to change.

Sensory processing differences, once considered specific to autism, are now recognized as common in ADHD as well. Research indicates that 40-60% of individuals with ADHD experience sensory processing difficulties that may include hypersensitivity to environmental stimuli, sensory seeking behaviours, or difficulties filtering irrelevant sensory information (Little et al., 2018). These sensory features can closely resemble those seen in autism, though they may differ in their specific pattern and impact on behaviour.

Sensory Processing Differences in Autism and ADHD: Overlap and Distinction

In autism, sensory sensitivities often have a more pervasive impact on daily functioning and more directly drive restricted and repetitive behaviours such as covering ears, avoiding certain food textures, or seeking specific sensory experiences. In ADHD, sensory issues may manifest more as distractibility by environmental stimuli or sensory seeking behaviours that reflect general self-stimulation rather than the specific, consistent sensory patterns often seen in autism.

The co-occurrence of these conditions is remarkably high, with research consistently demonstrating bidirectional overlap. Studies suggest that 30-80% of individuals with autism show clinically significant ADHD symptoms, while approximately 20-50% of individuals with ADHD meet criteria for autism (Antshel & Russo, 2019). This frequent co-occurrence likely reflects shared genetic factors and neurobiological mechanisms, suggesting that these conditions represent different manifestations of partially overlapping neurodevelopmental differences rather than entirely distinct disorders.

Current research in genetics and neuroscience increasingly supports a dimensional view of neurodevelopmental conditions, where autism and ADHD represent different expressions of related neurobiological variations rather than categorically separate entities. As noted by Lichtenstein et al. (2010), "*genetic factors that influence autism also influence ADHD*" (p.1357). This understanding has important implications for assessment, suggesting that clinicians should be alert to features of both conditions rather than seeking to attribute all symptoms to a single diagnosis.

Historical diagnostic approaches treated autism and ADHD as mutually exclusive, with earlier versions of diagnostic systems explicitly stating that ADHD could not be diagnosed in the presence of autism. This exclusionary criterion reflected the assumption that ADHD symptoms in autistic individuals were better explained by autism itself rather than representing a distinct co-occurring condition. Current diagnostic frameworks in both DSM-5 and ICD-11 have removed this exclusion, recognizing that these conditions commonly co-occur and that individuals may benefit from interventions targeting both conditions (Mahajan et al., 2012).

Despite the extensive overlap, several distinguishing features can help differentiate between autism and ADHD when they present separately, and identify their co-occurrence when both are present:

Primary attention deficits versus selective attention based on interest represents a key distinction in attentional patterns. In ADHD, attention difficulties are generally pervasive, affecting focus across most contexts, though they may improve somewhat during high-interest or novel activities. This pattern reflects a fundamental difficulty with attention regulation regardless of content. In autism, attention is often extremely focused and sustained for preferred interests or activities, while being significantly reduced for non-preferred tasks. This pattern of selective attention in autism reflects intense focus on topics of interest rather than general difficulties with attention regulation (Geurts et al., 2009).

During assessment, it's important to explore not just whether attention difficulties exist but their pattern across different contexts and activities: "Are there some activities where you can focus very well for long periods?" "What kinds of things capture and hold your attention easily?" "Do you sometimes focus so intensely on interests that you lose track of time or forget other responsibilities?" Individuals with autism often describe a stark contrast between their ability to focus on preferred versus non-preferred activities, while those with ADHD typically report more consistent attention challenges despite interest level.

Impulsivity versus social disinhibition reflects different mechanisms underlying similar behaviours. In ADHD, impulsivity stems from difficulties with response inhibition that affect behaviour across contexts. Individuals with ADHD often act or speak without thinking, make decisions impulsively, struggle with delayed gratification, and have difficulty restraining automatic responses regardless of the situation. In autism, apparent impulsivity in social situations often reflects misunderstanding of social norms or difficulties with perspective-taking rather than general inhibitory control problems. Individuals with autism may speak bluntly about sensitive topics, interrupt to discuss their interests, or behave in socially unexpected ways because they don't intuitively understand the social rules rather than because they cannot inhibit known inappropriate responses (Antshel et al., 2016).

These different mechanisms may produce similar observable behaviours, such as interrupting conversations or making socially inappropriate comments, but their underlying causes differ. Assessment should explore the consistency of disinhibited behaviour across contexts and the individual's awareness of social expectations: "*Do you find yourself acting without thinking across many situations, or primarily in social contexts?*" "*Are you aware of social rules but have trouble stopping yourself from breaking them, or do you sometimes realize only afterward that what you said or did wasn't appropriate?*" Individuals with ADHD often report knowing what they should do but acting before they can stop themselves, while those with autism may describe confusion about why their behaviour was inappropriate or difficulty predicting how others would react.

Hyperactivity versus repetitive movements involves different patterns of motor activity. The hyperactivity characteristic of ADHD typically involves general restlessness, fidgeting, and difficulty remaining still or quiet, often in response to feelings of internal restlessness or a need to release energy. This motor activity tends to be variable in presentation rather than following specific patterns. Repetitive movements in autism, such as hand-flapping, rocking, or complex finger movements, are typically more patterned and specific, often serving sensory or self-regulatory functions rather than reflecting general motor restlessness. These movements frequently occur in response to particular emotional states or sensory experiences and follow consistent patterns specific to the individual (Goldman et al., 2009).

Careful observation and questioning about the nature, triggers, and function of motor movements can help distinguish between these patterns: "*What kinds of physical movements do you find yourself doing when sitting still for long periods?*" "*What triggers these movements?*" "*How do these movements make you feel?*" "*Do you have specific movements that you repeat in particular situations?*" The responses may reveal important qualitative differences in the nature and purpose of motor activity.

The assessment of adults with possible autism, ADHD, or both conditions requires a comprehensive approach that examines not only current symptoms but developmental history, contextual factors, and functional impact. Several specific assessment strategies are particularly valuable:

Specific ADHD measures provide structured evaluation of attention, hyperactivity, and impulsivity symptoms across the lifespan. The **Diagnostic Interview for ADHD in Adults (DIVA)** offers a comprehensive interview format exploring both current and childhood symptoms across attention, hyperactivity, and impulsivity domains. The **Adult ADHD Self-Report Scale (ASRS)** provides an efficient screening tool validated for identifying adult ADHD. These measures help determine whether attention and hyperactivity symptoms are present at a clinically significant level, independent of autism features.

Detailed developmental history is essential, as both conditions are neurodevelopmental in origin but may show different patterns of early features. Assessment should explore:

1. Early attention patterns, activity level, and impulse control
2. Development of social communication, reciprocity, and play
3. Presence of restricted interests, repetitive behaviours, or sensory sensitivities in childhood
4. Family history of both conditions, given their strong genetic components
5. Developmental trajectory of symptoms across different contexts and developmental stages
6. Educational history, including specific challenges and accommodations
7. Response to previous interventions, including any medication trials

When features of both conditions are present in the developmental history, co-occurrence is more likely than when one set of features emerges much later than the other.

Response to structure and routine provides informative clinical data, as individuals with ADHD and autism often respond differently to environmental structure. Those with ADHD typically benefit from externally imposed structure but may struggle to create and maintain it themselves. Structure often helps compensate for executive functioning difficulties, supporting attention and task completion. Individuals with autism often create and adhere to their own routines and may become distressed when these routines are disrupted, reflecting the need for predictability and sameness characteristic of autism. While both groups benefit from structure, the relationship to structure and routine differs in quality.

Assessment should explore both the individual's need for structure and their response when routines are changed or interrupted.

Medication response, when available, can provide additional diagnostic information. Stimulant medications and other ADHD-specific pharmacological treatments typically improve core ADHD symptoms of attention, hyperactivity, and impulsivity but do not significantly affect autism features such as social communication differences or restricted and repetitive behaviours. If the individual has previously received ADHD medication, exploring which symptoms improved and which remained unchanged can help clarify the diagnostic picture. However, medication response should never be used as the sole basis for diagnosis, as individual responses vary considerably.

When features of both autism and ADHD are present at clinically significant levels, current best practice supports diagnosing both conditions rather than attempting to attribute all symptoms to one diagnosis. This approach, aligned with current ICD-11 and DSM-5 frameworks, acknowledges the frequent co-occurrence of these conditions and ensures that individuals receive appropriate interventions targeting all relevant areas of difficulty.

The practical implications of accurately identifying autism, ADHD, or their co-occurrence are significant and directly impact support planning:

1. Intervention approaches differ, with ADHD treatments focusing on medication, behavioural strategies for attention and executive functioning, and environmental modifications, while autism interventions emphasize social communication skills, environmental adaptations for sensory needs, and support for managing change and transitions. When both conditions co-occur, comprehensive intervention addressing both sets of needs is optimal.
2. Educational and workplace accommodations may differ based on the specific profile of strengths and challenges associated with each condition or their combination. ADHD accommodations often focus on reducing distractions, breaking tasks into manageable chunks, providing external organization systems, and allowing movement breaks. Autism accommodations more typically address sensory environment, social expectations, communication supports, and predictability. Accurate diagnosis helps ensure appropriate accommodations that address the individual's actual needs.
3. Self-understanding is enhanced by accurate diagnosis that explains the individual's lived experience. Many adults report that understanding the relationship between autism and ADHD features in their own presentation

provides significant clarification of lifelong patterns and challenges. This understanding can reduce self-blame, improve self-advocacy, and guide personal development of coping strategies.

The differentiation and identification of co-occurring autism and ADHD represents one of the most common and complex diagnostic challenges in adult autism assessment. It requires clinical sophistication, comprehensive assessment across multiple domains, and careful integration of information from various sources. When conducted thoroughly, this process leads to diagnostic clarity that forms the foundation for effective, personalized intervention planning.

CHAPTER 23

Differential Diagnosis - Anxiety Disorders

Anxiety disorders frequently overlap with autism spectrum disorder in both presentation and co-occurrence, creating significant challenges for differential diagnosis. Understanding the complex relationship between anxiety and autism is essential for accurate assessment and effective intervention planning. While anxiety disorders represent the most common co-occurring mental health conditions in autism—with lifetime prevalence rates of 50-70%—they can also present with features that mimic autism or mask its underlying presentation.

Social Anxiety Disorder (SAD)

Social Anxiety Disorder (SAD) shares particularly significant overlap with the social communication domain of autism, as both conditions involve difficulties with social interaction and potential avoidance of social situations. However, the underlying mechanisms driving these social difficulties differ substantially between the conditions.

Fear and avoidance versus lack of social understanding represents a key distinction. In SAD, social difficulties stem primarily from fear of negative evaluation, embarrassment, or rejection, rather than from fundamental difficulties understanding social dynamics. Individuals with SAD typically possess adequate social knowledge and skills but experience intense anxiety that interferes with their execution. In contrast, the social difficulties in autism reflect more fundamental differences in social cognition, pragmatic language, and nonverbal communication that exist independent of anxiety, though anxiety may certainly exacerbate these challenges.

Assessment should explore not only the presence of social avoidance but its underlying motivations and the individual's social understanding: " *What concerns you about social situations?" "Do you understand what's expected in social situations but feel too anxious to do it, or do you sometimes feel confused about what's expected?" "If you could interact without feeling anxious, would you know how to behave appropriately?"* Individuals with primary SAD typically report understanding social expectations but feeling too anxious to meet them, while those with autism often describe fundamental confusion about social rules or dynamics.

Preservation of social skills in non-threatening contexts provides another important distinction. Individuals with SAD often demonstrate intact social communication skills in safe, comfortable environments or with familiar people where anxiety is minimal. Their social difficulties typically fluctuate based on their anxiety level and the perceived evaluative threat of the situation. In contrast, the social communication differences in autism tend to be more consistent across contexts, though they may be more or less apparent depending on environmental demands and supports.

Assessment should examine social functioning across various contexts: "*Are there some social situations where you feel comfortable and can interact easily?*" "*How does your social comfort and performance differ between familiar and unfamiliar settings?*" "*How has your social functioning changed over time or with treatment for anxiety?*" Individuals with primary SAD often identify specific contexts where they can interact effectively, while those with autism typically report more pervasive social differences despite varying anxiety levels.

Physiological anxiety symptoms often provide additional diagnostic information. SAD typically involves prominent physical symptoms of anxiety during social situations, including racing heart, sweating, trembling, blushing, nausea, or panic attacks. While individuals with autism may also experience anxiety symptoms in social settings, especially if they have co-occurring SAD, their social difficulties persist even when anxiety is well-managed. Assessment should explore both the presence of physical anxiety symptoms during social interaction and the relationship between anxiety management and social functioning.

The assessment approach should consider several additional factors when differentiating between autism and anxiety disorders:

Anxiety-specific measures such as the **Generalized Anxiety Disorder-7 (GAD-7), Liebowitz Social Anxiety Scale (LSAS),** or **Yale-Brown Obsessive Compulsive Scale (Y-BOCS)** provide structured assessment of specific anxiety symptoms and their severity. These measures help determine whether anxiety symptoms reach clinical significance and clarify their relationship to social and behavioural patterns.

Exploring the function of repetitive behaviours provides important differential diagnostic information. In autism, restricted and repetitive behaviours often serve various functions, including self-regulation, sensory stimulation, or expression of interests, and are typically experienced as comfortable, calming, or pleasurable.

In anxiety disorders, particularly **Obsessive-Compulsive Disorder (OCD)**, repetitive behaviours primarily function to reduce anxiety and prevent feared outcomes, and are often experienced as unwanted or distressing.

Assessment should explore the subjective experience of repetitive behaviours: "*How do you feel when engaging in these behaviours?*" "*What happens if you're prevented from doing them?*" "*Do these behaviours feel pleasurable or distressing?*" "*Do they happen more when you're anxious, or consistently regardless of your anxiety level?*" The responses often reveal qualitatively different experiences between autism-related and anxiety-driven repetitive behaviours.

Developmental trajectory of symptoms provides crucial context for differential diagnosis. Autism features typically emerge in early development, with social communication differences and restricted, repetitive behaviours present from childhood, though they may become more apparent or impairing as social demands increase with age. Anxiety disorders more commonly emerge later in development, often in late childhood, adolescence, or early adulthood, though they can certainly occur earlier.

Careful developmental history should explore the timing and evolution of both social communication difficulties and anxiety symptoms: "*When did you first start experiencing difficulties in social situations?*" "*Have you always felt uncomfortable or confused in social settings, or did this develop at a particular time?*" "*When did you first notice anxiety symptoms, and how have they changed over time?*" This developmental perspective helps distinguish between lifelong neurodevelopmental differences and later-emerging anxiety disorders.

Co-occurrence of anxiety and autism is extremely common, requiring sophisticated assessment that can identify both conditions when present. The high prevalence of anxiety in autism likely reflects multiple factors:

1. Inherent challenges of navigating a social world with different neurocognitive processing
2. Repeated experiences of social rejection, misunderstanding, or failure
3. Sensory sensitivities that create ongoing environmental stress
4. Difficulty with unpredictability and change
5. Potential shared neurobiological mechanisms
6. Heightened awareness of difference, particularly in individuals diagnosed later in life

When both conditions co-exist, a comprehensive formulation should address how they interact and influence each other. For example, core autism features may create ongoing social challenges that generate anxiety, while anxiety may then further impair social functioning or exacerbate restricted and repetitive behaviours, creating a reinforcing cycle that requires intervention addressing both conditions.

Obsessive-Compulsive Disorder (OCD) shares particular overlap with the restricted and repetitive behaviour domain of autism, as both conditions may involve ritualized behaviours, intense preoccupations, and resistance to change. However, several key distinctions help differentiate between these presentations:

Ego-dystonic rituals versus preferred routines reflects a fundamental difference in the subjective experience of repetitive behaviours. In OCD, compulsions are typically experienced as unwanted and distressing—performed not for inherent enjoyment but to neutralize anxiety or prevent feared outcomes. The individual generally recognizes these behaviours as excessive or unreasonable but feels unable to stop them. In contrast, the routines and repetitive behaviours in autism are often experienced as comfortable, pleasurable, or simply preferred. They typically feel ego-syntonic (aligned with the person's sense of self) rather than imposed by anxiety.

Assessment should explore the subjective experience of routines and rituals: "How do you feel about these behaviours?" "Would you continue them if you had the choice, or would you prefer to stop?" "Do these behaviours cause distress, or do they help you feel better?" Individuals with OCD typically report wishing they could stop their compulsions despite feeling driven to perform them, while those with autism often describe their routines as positive or necessary for their well-being.

Content of obsessions provides another important distinction. In OCD, obsessions typically focus on specific themes such as contamination, harm, symmetry, or taboo thoughts. These obsessions generate anxiety that is temporarily relieved by compulsive behaviours. In autism, preoccupations usually involve intense interests in specific topics, systems, or objects, approached with enthusiasm rather than anxiety. While these interests may sometimes appear unusual in content or intensity, they differ qualitatively from the intrusive, distressing thoughts characteristic of OCD.

Assessment should explore the nature of preoccupations: "*What kinds of thoughts occupy your mind most often?*" "*Are these thoughts pleasant or unpleasant?*" "*Do you deliberately think about these topics because you enjoy them, or do the thoughts intrude against your will?*" The responses typically reveal qualitatively different thought patterns between autism-related interests and OCD obsessions.

Response to exposure therapy offers additional diagnostic information when available. OCD typically responds to specific cognitive-behavioural interventions, particularly exposure and response prevention (ERP), which involves gradually facing feared situations without performing compulsions. The restricted and repetitive behaviours in autism generally do not show the same pattern of response to ERP, as they are not primarily maintained by anxiety reduction.

When exposure-based approaches have been attempted, exploring the response can be informative: *"What happened when you tried to resist these behaviours?" "Did your anxiety decrease over time with repeated exposure, or did preventing the behaviours continue to cause distress?"* The pattern of response often differs significantly between OCD compulsions and autism-related repetitive behaviours.

The assessment approach for differentiating anxiety disorders from autism should be comprehensive, integrating information from multiple sources:

1. Standardized autism measures, particularly those examining restricted and repetitive behaviours
2. Anxiety-specific measures assessing various dimensions of anxiety
3. Detailed developmental history exploring the emergence and evolution of both autism features and anxiety symptoms
4. Functional analysis of repetitive behaviours, examining their triggers, subjective experience, and consequences
5. Response to previous interventions, particularly anxiety-focused treatments
6. Collateral information from others who know the individual across different contexts and developmental periods

This multi-method assessment approach provides the most reliable basis for distinguishing between autism, anxiety disorders, and their common co-occurrence. When both conditions are present, accurate identification of each ensures that intervention planning addresses the full range of the individual's needs.

Practical implications for support and treatment differ significantly based on the diagnostic formulation:

1. Primary anxiety disorders typically respond well to evidence-based psychological interventions such as cognitive-behavioural therapy and, in some cases, psychopharmacological approaches
2. Autism features require different support approaches focused on understanding and accommodating neurodevelopmental differences rather than treating them as symptoms to be eliminated
3. When both conditions co-occur, integrated intervention approaches that address both anxiety management and autism-specific needs yield the best outcomes

Accurate differential diagnosis between autism and anxiety disorders, or recognition of their co-occurrence, provides the foundation for personalized intervention planning that effectively addresses the individual's unique pattern of strengths and challenges.

CHAPTER 24
Comorbidity Assessment

Comprehensive autism assessment must include thorough evaluation of potential co-occurring conditions, as adults with autism experience significantly higher rates of both mental health and physical health comorbidities compared to the general population. These co-occurring conditions often have substantial impacts on functioning and quality of life, sometimes creating more significant impairment than core autism features themselves. Identifying and addressing comorbidities is therefore essential for developing effective support plans and improving outcomes for adults with autism.

Mental health comorbidities occur at strikingly high rates in the autistic population. Understanding these patterns of co-occurrence, their presentation in the context of autism, and appropriate assessment approaches is crucial for comprehensive clinical care.

Depression represents one of the most common co-occurring conditions, with lifetime prevalence estimates of approximately 40% in adults with autism—several times higher than general population rates. This elevated prevalence likely reflects multiple factors, including:

1. Neurobiological vulnerabilities that may increase susceptibility to mood disorders
2. Chronic stress from navigating a social world designed for different neurotypes
3. Higher rates of negative life experiences such as bullying, social rejection, and unemployment
4. Greater difficulty accessing appropriate mental health support
5. The impact of late diagnosis and years of "camouflaging" or attempting to appear neurotypical

The presentation of depression may differ in autism, creating assessment challenges. Traditional symptoms such as social withdrawal, reduced communication, or changes in routine may be difficult to distinguish from autism features or may manifest differently in autistic individuals. Additionally, alexithymia (difficulty identifying and describing emotions), which is common in autism, may make it harder for individuals to recognize and report mood symptoms.

Assessment should incorporate autism-informed approaches to depression screening, including:

1. Concrete questioning about specific symptoms rather than abstract questions about mood
2. Attention to changes from the individual's baseline rather than comparison to typical presentations
3. Exploration of possible behavioural equivalents of depressed mood, such as increased irritability, sensory sensitivity, or repetitive behaviours
4. Collateral information from those who know the individual well and can identify subtle mood changes
5. Consideration of validated depression measures specifically adapted for autism when available

Anxiety disorders occur in 50-70% of adults with autism, making them the most common co-occurring mental health conditions. This category includes generalized anxiety disorder, social anxiety disorder, specific phobias, panic disorder, and agoraphobia, all of which occur at elevated rates in autistic populations. As with depression, multiple factors likely contribute to this high prevalence, including inherent challenges navigating unpredictable social and sensory environments, negative life experiences, and potentially shared neurobiological mechanisms.

Anxiety may present atypically in autism, with features such as:

1. Increased repetitive behaviours rather than typical worry statements
2. Sensory sensitivities that intensify during periods of anxiety
3. Behavioural difficulties, shutdown, or meltdowns rather than verbal expression of anxiety
4. Concrete, specific fears rather than more generalized worry
5. Difficulty identifying and communicating the internal experience of anxiety

Assessment approaches should adapt to these potential differences, incorporating:

1. Functional analysis of behaviours that may represent anxiety equivalents
2. Careful differentiation between social communication difficulties inherent to autism and those driven by social anxiety

3. Exploration of the relationship between routines, resistance to change, and anxiety management
4. Both self-report and observer-report measures of anxiety symptoms
5. Consideration of how sensory sensitivities might interact with anxiety symptoms

Obsessive-Compulsive Disorder (OCD) affects approximately 20% of adults with autism—a rate significantly higher than the general population. The distinction between autism-related restricted and repetitive behaviours and OCD compulsions can be challenging but is crucial for appropriate intervention planning.

Assessment should focus on:

1. The function and subjective experience of repetitive behaviours (ego-dystonic distress in OCD versus comfort or interest in autism)
2. The presence of specific obsessions driving compulsive behaviours in OCD
3. The relationship between anxiety and repetitive behaviours
4. Changes in the pattern or intensity of repetitive behaviours over time
5. Response to previous interventions, particularly exposure-based approaches

ADHD co-occurs in 30-50% of adults with autism, creating complex clinical presentations that require careful assessment of attention, activity level, and impulse control separate from autism features. The previously discussed approaches to differential diagnosis apply equally to comorbidity assessment, with emphasis on identifying when both conditions are present rather than attempting to attribute all symptoms to a single diagnosis.

Neurodevelopmental comorbidities beyond ADHD also occur at elevated rates in the autistic population and warrant specific assessment:

Intellectual disability co-occurs in approximately 30% of individuals with autism, though this rate may be lower in adult populations presenting for first-time assessment, as individuals with both conditions are more likely to be identified earlier in life. When intellectual disability is suspected, formal cognitive assessment is essential for diagnostic clarification and support planning. Autism assessment must be adapted to the individual's cognitive level, with greater emphasis on observation and informant report rather than self-report measures when intellectual disability is present.

Specific learning disorders such as dyslexia, dyscalculia, and dysgraphia occur at higher rates in autism and may contribute significantly to academic

and occupational challenges. Assessment should explore educational history for indications of specific learning difficulties, potentially including formal psychoeducational assessment when indicated. Identifying specific learning disorders allows for targeted educational accommodations and support strategies that address these challenges separately from autism-specific needs.

Developmental coordination disorder (DCD), characterized by motor coordination difficulties that significantly impact functioning, co-occurs in 30-50% of individuals with autism. These motor challenges may affect handwriting, self-care skills, sports participation, and various daily living activities. Assessment should include exploration of motor development history and current motor coordination challenges, with referral for specialized occupational therapy assessment when significant difficulties are identified.

Medical comorbidities occur at elevated rates in autism and may significantly impact quality of life, functioning, and presentation of autism features. Comprehensive assessment should include screening for common co-occurring medical conditions:

Epilepsy affects approximately 20-30% of individuals with autism, with risk varying based on presence of intellectual disability and other factors. Seizures may sometimes be subtle or atypical in presentation. Assessment should include careful history of possible seizure activity, particularly episodes of apparent "zoning out," unusual sensory experiences, or unexplained periods of altered awareness. When seizures are suspected, referral for neurological evaluation is essential.

Sleep disorders are extremely common in autism, with 50-80% of individuals experiencing significant sleep problems including delayed sleep onset, frequent night wakings, early morning awakening, or irregular sleep patterns. These difficulties likely reflect multiple factors including circadian rhythm differences, sensory sensitivities, anxiety, and potential neurobiological differences in sleep regulation. Assessment should thoroughly explore sleep patterns, their impact on functioning, and potential contributing factors. Addressing sleep problems can significantly improve overall functioning and reduce other symptoms.

Gastrointestinal issues occur in 30-70% of individuals with autism, including conditions such as irritable bowel syndrome, constipation, diarrhoea, food intolerances, and reflux. These issues may be underreported due to communication differences or interoceptive challenges that make it difficult to identify and describe internal sensations. Assessment should specifically inquire about gastrointestinal symptoms, dietary patterns, and their potential relationship to behavioural or emotional presentation, as untreated gastrointestinal problems can significantly impact comfort, behaviour, and participation in daily activities.

Genetic syndromes associated with autism should be considered when certain clinical features are present. Conditions such as Fragile X syndrome, Tuberous Sclerosis Complex, Rett syndrome, and various chromosomal variations occur at higher rates in autism and may have specific medical implications. Assessment should include medical history, family history, and physical examination for features suggestive of genetic conditions, with referral for genetic consultation when indicated. Identifying specific genetic conditions can provide important information about associated medical risks, developmental course, and potential interventions.

The assessment approach for comorbidities should be systematic and comprehensive, recognizing that:

1. Symptoms may present atypically in the context of autism
2. Communication differences may affect symptom reporting
3. Different comorbidities may interact with each other and with core autism features
4. The presence of comorbidities significantly impacts intervention planning and prognosis

Structured screening followed by detailed assessment represents an efficient approach to comorbidity evaluation. Initial screening may include:

1. Brief standardized measures for common mental health conditions
2. Review of systems for medical symptoms
3. Developmental and educational history for neurodevelopmental comorbidities
4. Family history for conditions with genetic components

When screening suggests potential comorbidities, more detailed assessment should follow, potentially including:

1. Condition-specific diagnostic measures
2. Consultation with specialists in relevant areas
3. Medical investigations when indicated
4. Functional analysis of how comorbid symptoms interact with autism features

The integration of comorbidity assessment with autism diagnostic evaluation requires clinical sophistication and a dimensional approach that recognizes the complex interactions between autism and co-occurring conditions. Rather than viewing comorbidities as separate, distinct entities, assessment should explore how they intertwine with and potentially amplify autism features, creating unique clinical presentations that require individualized intervention approaches.

For example, anxiety may increase sensory sensitivities and repetitive behaviours, which in turn may further increase anxiety in challenging environments. Sleep problems may exacerbate executive functioning difficulties and emotional dysregulation. ADHD symptoms may amplify the social communication challenges associated with autism by adding difficulties with attention to social cues and impulse control in social situations.

Understanding these complex interactions forms the foundation for comprehensive support planning that addresses the individual's complete clinical picture rather than focusing solely on autism features. This integrated approach ultimately leads to more effective interventions and improved quality of life for adults with autism and co-occurring conditions.

CHAPTER 25

ASD with Intellectual Disability

The assessment of autism spectrum disorder in adults with intellectual disability presents distinct challenges that require specific adaptations to standard assessment approaches. Approximately 30% of individuals with autism have co-occurring **intellectual disability (ID),** defined as significant limitations in both intellectual functioning (IQ below 70) and adaptive behaviour with onset during the developmental period. While this co-occurrence rate is lower than historical estimates—reflecting improved recognition of autism in individuals without ID—it remains a common and clinically important presentation that requires specialized assessment expertise.

The prevalence of autism is significantly higher in populations with **intellectual disability** than in the general population. Research suggests that 10-40% of individuals with ID meet criteria for autism, with higher rates associated with more severe levels of intellectual disability. This bidirectional relationship likely reflects shared genetic and neurodevelopmental pathways between these conditions. In clinical practice, this means that adults with ID should be considered at higher risk for undiagnosed autism, particularly when social communication difficulties or restricted and repetitive behaviours are present.

Assessment challenges in this population are numerous and require thoughtful adaptations to standard approaches:

Communication limitations affecting self-report represent a primary challenge, as many standardized autism assessment tools rely heavily on verbal self-report or require significant language comprehension. Individuals with ID may have limited expressive language, receptive language difficulties, or both, reducing the validity of standard self-report measures and structured interviews. This challenge necessitates greater reliance on observational assessment, informant report, and behavioural history to gather diagnostic information.

Adapting communication during assessment is essential and may include:

1. Using simpler language and concrete questions
2. Providing visual supports to complement verbal information

3. Allowing additional time for processing and responding
4. Checking comprehension through demonstration rather than asking "Do you understand?"
5. Being attentive to non-verbal forms of communication including behaviour, facial expression, and vocalizations
6. Working with familiar communication partners who can interpret idiosyncratic communication

Adaptations needed for standardized assessments depend on the individual's level of intellectual and communication functioning. For individuals with mild ID who have functional language, standard instruments may be usable with modifications such as simplified language, additional examples, or extended time. For those with moderate to severe ID or limited language, alternative approaches are necessary:

Observational scales such as the **ADOS-2 Module 1 or 2** (designed for individuals with limited language) may be appropriate, though even these may require adaptation for adults, as they were primarily developed for children. The administration should focus on creating appropriate social presses and opportunities for observation while being flexible about the specific activities used to engage the individual.

Informant-based assessments become particularly important when direct assessment is limited by communication or cognitive factors. Measures specifically designed for individuals with intellectual disability and possible autism include:

1. The **Diagnostic Assessment for the Severely Handicapped, Revised (DASH-II):** Screens for psychiatric conditions, including autism, in individuals with severe and profound ID
2. The **Pervasive Developmental Disorder in Mental Retardation Scale (PDD-MRS):** Specifically assesses autism features in individuals with ID
3. The **Autism Spectrum Disorders-Diagnosis for Intellectually Disabled Adults (ASD-DA)**: Designed specifically for diagnosing autism in adults with intellectual disability
4. Adapted versions of standard measures such as the **Social Communication Questionnaire (SCQ)** or the **Autism Spectrum Quotient (AQ),** though these should be used with caution as their validation in adult ID populations may be limited

Functional behaviour analysis provides valuable assessment information by examining the antecedents, behaviours, and consequences of specific behavioural patterns. This approach is particularly useful for understanding behaviours that might reflect autism features, such as repetitive movements, sensory-seeking behaviours, or social avoidance. By systematically analysing the contexts in which behaviours occur and their apparent functions, clinicians can better distinguish between behaviours related to autism and those better explained by other factors such as communication limitations, environmental stressors, or learned patterns.

Distinguishing ASD-specific behaviours from ID-related behaviours represents perhaps the most significant challenge in this population. Several behavioural features commonly occur in ID independent of autism but may superficially resemble autism features:

1. Self-stimulatory behaviours and stereotyped movements often occur in ID without autism, particularly at lower developmental levels or in restrictive environments with limited stimulation. Assessment should explore whether these behaviours:
    - Occur across different contexts or primarily when unstimulated
    - Show the specific, consistent patterns more characteristic of autism
    - Persist despite environmental enrichment and skill development
    - Serve specific sensory or regulatory functions versus general stimulation
2. Social communication differences in ID without autism typically align with overall developmental level and improve with developmental progress. In contrast, the social communication differences in autism often show a distinct pattern of strengths and challenges that is inconsistent with overall development. Assessment should consider whether social communication:
    - Is consistent with developmental level across domains
    - Shows specific qualitative differences beyond what would be expected based on cognitive functioning
    - Includes atypical nonverbal communication such as unusual eye contact or facial expression
    - Demonstrates better rote social skills than social understanding
3. Restricted interests may be difficult to evaluate in ID, as overall interests may be limited by cognitive level, exposure, and opportunity. Assessment should explore whether interests:
    - Are unusual in intensity and focus compared to others at similar developmental levels
    - Interfere with broader skill development and experiences

- Have the repetitive, systematic quality characteristic of autism special interests
- Persist despite opportunities for broader engagement

Developmental history takes on particular importance in differentiating autism from ID alone, as the developmental trajectory may reveal autism-specific patterns beyond general developmental delay. Assessment should explore:

1. Early social communication milestones relative to general development
2. Patterns of play and social interest in childhood
3. Development of joint attention, social referencing, and shared enjoyment
4. Emergence of repetitive behaviours and sensory differences
5. Response to social and communication interventions over time

Diagnostic Overshadowing in Individuals with Intellectual Disability

Diagnostic overshadowing—the tendency to attribute all behavioural or emotional symptoms to ID rather than recognizing additional conditions—represents a significant risk in this population. This can lead to missed autism diagnoses when social, communication, or behavioural differences are simply attributed to intellectual disability without considering whether they show the specific pattern characteristic of autism. Thorough assessment guards against diagnostic overshadowing by systematically evaluating autism-specific features while accounting for developmental level.

UK service considerations for adults with co-occurring autism and ID include the question of whether these individuals are best served by integrated or separate ID and autism services. Current practice varies across regions, with several models in operation:

1. Integrated neurodevelopmental services that address both autism and ID within a single team
2. Intellectual disability services with embedded autism expertise
3. Autism services that extend to individuals with co-occurring ID
4. Collaborative approaches where autism and ID services work together for individuals with both conditions

Each model has advantages and limitations, but all require clinicians with specific expertise in assessing and supporting individuals with co-occurring conditions. Best practice involves person-centred approaches that address the individual's unique combination of support needs regardless of service structure.

Assessment adaptations for adults with ID should consider several additional factors:

1. Physical health conditions that may impact behaviour or presentation
2. Medication effects that might influence social engagement or behaviour
3. Environmental factors, including restrictive settings that may limit opportunities for social interaction or increase repetitive behaviour's
4. Trauma history, as individuals with ID experience higher rates of adverse experiences that may affect behaviour and emotional presentation
5. Communication method and history, including any augmentative and alternative communication approaches

The diagnostic decision-making process should integrate information from multiple sources while considering developmental level. When determining whether an adult with ID meets criteria for autism, clinicians should:

1. Compare social communication and behaviour to what would be expected at the individual's developmental level rather than chronological age
2. Look for the specific pattern of social communication differences characteristic of autism, beyond general delays
3. Consider whether restricted and repetitive behaviour's show the quality and function associated with autism rather than simply reflecting developmental level
4. Evaluate the consistency of autism features across different contexts and with different people
5. Assess the developmental trajectory for patterns consistent with autism rather than ID alone

Functional impact assessment is particularly important, as it guides support planning regardless of diagnostic conclusions. This assessment should explore:

1. How potential autism features affect the individual's quality of life
2. Whether specific autism-focused supports might benefit the individual
3. Environmental adaptations that could enhance functioning and well-being
4. Strategies for supporting communication and social engagement at the individual's developmental level

The formulation and feedback process should emphasize practical implications for support rather than focusing exclusively on diagnostic classification. For many adults with ID, the most valuable outcome of assessment is a detailed understanding of their individual pattern of strengths, challenges, and support needs, which informs person-centred planning regardless of whether formal autism criteria are met.

When working with adults with co-occurring ID and autism, assessment represents the foundation for comprehensive support planning that addresses both conditions and their interaction. Effective support typically includes:

1. Communication approaches adapted to the individual's specific profile
2. Environmental modifications addressing sensory needs and predictability
3. Structured teaching of functional and social skills
4. Positive behaviour support strategies for challenging behaviour's
5. Meaningful activity and community participation opportunities
6. Support for families and carers to understand and respond to the individual's unique needs

By conducting thorough, adapted assessment that recognizes both the challenges and strengths associated with co-occurring autism and intellectual disability, clinicians provide the foundation for support planning that enhances quality of life and promotes optimal development and independence.

CHAPTER 26

ASD without Intellectual Disability

Autism spectrum disorder without intellectual disability represents a distinct clinical presentation that requires specific assessment considerations and approaches. This presentation—historically classified as Asperger's syndrome or high-functioning autism—involves the core social communication differences and restricted, repetitive behaviour patterns characteristic of autism, but without the significant limitations in intellectual functioning that define intellectual disability. Understanding the specific features, assessment challenges, and support needs of this population is essential for effective clinical practice.

The historical context of autism without intellectual disability provides important perspective on current diagnostic approaches. In previous diagnostic systems, Asperger's syndrome was classified as a distinct condition characterized by qualitative differences in social interaction and restricted, repetitive patterns of behaviour, interests, and activities, without clinically significant general language delay or intellectual disability. This classification reflected Hans Asperger's original descriptions of children with marked social difficulties despite strong verbal and cognitive abilities.

The diagnostic landscape changed significantly with DSM-5 in 2013 and subsequently ICD-11, which removed Asperger's syndrome as a separate diagnosis and incorporated it within the broader autism spectrum disorder category. This change reflected growing research evidence that the boundaries between Asperger's syndrome and autism without language delay were not reliably distinguishable, with similar outcomes, neurobiological findings, and genetic factors across these previously separated conditions.

Current classification in **ICD-11** uses autism spectrum disorder without intellectual disability **(ICD-11 code 6A02.0)** as the diagnostic category for individuals who meet autism criteria but have IQ scores in the average range or above (generally IQ ≥ 70). This classification may be further specified based on functional language level, allowing for distinctions between individuals with and without language impairment. This dimensional approach recognizes the heterogeneity within autism while acknowledging that intellectual functioning represents an important specifier that influences presentation, support needs, and prognosis.

The transition away from Asperger's syndrome as a diagnostic label has generated considerable debate within both clinical and autistic communities. Many individuals diagnosed with Asperger's syndrome developed strong identity connections to this terminology and expressed concerns about its elimination. Others welcomed the move toward a unified spectrum concept that recognizes the fundamental similarities across different autism presentations. Clinicians should be sensitive to these perspectives when discussing diagnosis with adults, acknowledging the personal significance that specific terminology may hold while explaining current diagnostic frameworks.

Assessment considerations for autism without intellectual disability include several specific challenges and approaches:

Higher masking and camouflaging frequently characterize this presentation, particularly in adults who have developed sophisticated strategies to compensate for social communication differences. These compensatory strategies may include explicit learning of social rules, preparation of conversational scripts, imitation of others' social behaviour, and deliberate suppression of autism-related behaviours in social settings. This masking often makes autism features less obvious in brief clinical encounters or structured settings, potentially leading to missed or delayed diagnosis.

Assessment must be adapted to identify autism despite effective compensation by:

1. Creating varied assessment contexts that challenge compensation strategies, including both structured and unstructured social situations
2. Extending assessment over multiple sessions to observe performance as cognitive resources for maintaining compensation may become depleted
3. Specifically inquiring about the effort required for social interaction, experiences of social exhaustion, and differences in behaviour between public and private settings
4. Gathering collateral information from multiple sources who know the individual across different contexts and time periods
5. Paying careful attention to subtle qualitative differences in social communication that may persist despite general social competence

Subtler presentation of social communication difficulties is common in this population. Rather than obvious absence of social interaction or dramatic language differences, individuals with autism without intellectual disability often show more nuanced social communication features such as:

1. Difficulties with the pragmatic aspects of language despite strong vocabulary and grammar
2. Challenges with the reciprocal nature of conversation, such as topic maintenance, turn-taking, and adjusting to the listener's interests and knowledge
3. Concrete or literal interpretation of language, with difficulty understanding implied meanings, metaphors, or humour
4. Subtle differences in prosody, facial expression, or gesture that affect the quality rather than the presence of nonverbal communication
5. Challenges with perspective-taking and theory of mind that become apparent primarily in complex social situations rather than simple social cognition tasks

Assessment must be sensitive to these subtler features, utilizing measures designed to capture higher-level social communication differences rather than basic social skills. Detailed conversation analysis, exploration of understanding of complex social scenarios, and assessment of pragmatic language use across contexts may reveal difficulties not apparent in more structured assessment components.

Sophisticated Special Interests in Autism Without Intellectual Disability

Sophisticated special interests represent another distinctive feature of autism without intellectual disability. Rather than obviously unusual or age-inappropriate interests, individuals in this population often develop intense, focused interests in topics that may appear age-appropriate or even professionally valuable but are pursued with unusual intensity, systematic focus, and attention to detail. These interests might include academic subjects, music, computer programming, creative writing, specific genres of literature or film, political activism, or historical periods.

Assessment should explore not only the content of interests but their quality and impact:

1. The intensity and focus with which interests are pursued
2. The systematic collection of information or objects related to the interest
3. The tendency to accumulate highly detailed knowledge within narrow domains
4. The degree to which interests may dominate conversation or time allocation

5. The extent to which interests might facilitate educational or occupational success versus potentially limiting broader development

Often diagnosis is later in this population, with many individuals not recognized as autistic until adolescence, adulthood, or even middle or later life. This delayed identification typically reflects a combination of factors:

1. Stronger cognitive and language abilities that compensate for or mask social difficulties
2. Development of effective camouflaging strategies that conceal autism features
3. Special interests that may facilitate educational or occupational success in specific niches
4. Historical limitations in professional understanding of how autism presents in individuals without intellectual disability, particularly females and those with stronger verbal abilities
5. Misdiagnosis with other conditions such as anxiety disorders, personality disorders, or mood disorders that may represent secondary features or co-occurring conditions

Late diagnosis has significant implications for the assessment process. Adults seeking assessment after decades of unrecognized autism often present with complex clinical pictures that include:

1. Secondary mental health conditions, particularly anxiety and depression, developed in response to chronic social challenges and the effort of camouflaging
2. Established compensatory strategies that may obscure classic autism presentations
3. Significant autobiographical insights about lifelong differences, which can be valuable for diagnosis but may also be influenced by research or reading about autism
4. A history of misdiagnoses, unsuccessful treatments, and accumulated psychological impact from not understanding the neurobiological basis of their differences

The assessment process must navigate these complexities, distinguishing between core autism features, secondary adaptations or conditions, and alternative explanations for the presenting difficulties.

Functional impact assessment is particularly important for this population, as the relationship between autism features and functional outcomes is highly variable in individuals without intellectual disability. Despite cognitive and language strengths, many adults with autism without intellectual disability experience significant challenges in multiple life domains:

Employment outcomes reveal concerning patterns, with studies consistently showing high rates of unemployment and underemployment relative to educational qualifications. Even when employed, many work in positions below their educational level or struggle with workplace social demands, sensory environments, executive functioning requirements, or adaptation to change. Assessment should explore not only employment status but job sustainability, workplace accommodations, and the fit between cognitive strengths and job requirements.

Independent living may present challenges despite strong intellectual abilities. Executive functioning difficulties affecting planning, organization, time management, and financial management can impact daily functioning. Sensory sensitivities may create difficulties with aspects of independent living such as shopping in busy environments, using public transportation, or managing household tasks with aversive sensory qualities. Assessment should examine both the capacity for independent living skills and the actual implementation of these skills in real-world contexts.

Relationships often represent an area of significant challenge. Many adults with autism without intellectual disability express interest in friendships and romantic relationships but struggle with their development and maintenance. Common difficulties include reading subtle social cues, understanding unstated relationship expectations, managing the sensory aspects of physical intimacy, and balancing relationship demands with personal needs for solitude or routine. Assessment should explore relationship history, current relationship status, satisfaction with relationships, and specific relationship challenges.

Mental health vulnerabilities are pronounced in this population, with exceptionally high rates of anxiety, depression, and suicidality compared to both the general population and individuals with autism and intellectual disability. These mental health challenges likely reflect multiple factors, including:

1. Chronic stress from navigating social demands with limited support or understanding
2. The psychological impact of camouflaging and suppressing natural behaviour's
3. Negative experiences such as bullying, rejection, or exploitation due to social vulnerabilities

4. Greater self-awareness of differences from peers, particularly during adolescence and young adulthood
5. Sensory and cognitive overwhelm in environments not designed for autistic neurotypes

Comprehensive assessment must include thorough evaluation of mental health status, history of mental health challenges, and their relationship to autism features and life experiences.

The assessment process for adults with suspected autism without intellectual disability should be tailored to this specific presentation:

1. Utilize assessment tools with sufficient sensitivity for subtler presentations, such as the ADOS-2 Module 4, which was designed specifically for verbally fluent adolescents and adults
2. Include measures of more complex social cognition rather than basic social skills
3. Employ detailed developmental interviewing that explores early indicators that may have been subtle or overlooked
4. Assess executive functioning in real-world contexts rather than relying solely on structured cognitive tasks
5. Explore the subjective experience of social interaction, including effort, stress, and compensatory strategies
6. Consider gender-based differences in presentation, as females with autism without intellectual disability may show particularly subtle or gender-specific features

The diagnostic decision-making process should integrate information across these multiple domains while considering the significant heterogeneity within autism without intellectual disability. Diagnostic conclusions should be accompanied by detailed formulation that captures the individual's unique profile of autism features, compensatory strategies, co-occurring conditions, and support needs.

Support recommendations must be individualized, recognizing that needs vary considerably despite similar diagnostic classifications. Effective support might include:

1. Psychoeducation about autism and its manifestations without intellectual disability
2. Strategies for managing sensory sensitivities in work, educational, and community environments

3. Disclosure decision-making support regarding if, when, and how to disclose autism in different contexts
4. Workplace or educational accommodations targeting specific needs while capitalizing on cognitive strengths
5. Social support strategies that respect individual preferences for social engagement while addressing specific social communication challenges
6. Executive functioning supports such as organizational systems, planning tools, or coaching
7. Mental health interventions adapted for autism when anxiety, depression, or other conditions co-occur

Through comprehensive assessment that recognizes both the challenges and strengths associated with autism without intellectual disability, clinicians can provide diagnostic clarity and support recommendations that significantly improve quality of life and functional outcomes for this population.

CHAPTER 27

Assessing Impact on Functioning

A comprehensive autism assessment must go beyond determining whether diagnostic criteria are met to examine how autism features impact the individual's functioning across various life domains. This functional impact assessment serves multiple purposes: it provides context for diagnostic decision-making, identifies specific areas where support may be beneficial, establishes a baseline for measuring the effectiveness of interventions, and helps determine eligibility for services and accommodations. For adults with autism, understanding the relationship between autism features and functional outcomes is essential for developing meaningful, person-centred support plans.

Educational history provides valuable insights into both historical and current functional impact of autism features. This exploration should extend beyond academic achievement to examine the broader educational experience across different stages and settings:

Academic achievements versus social experiences often show discrepancies in individuals with autism, particularly those without intellectual disabilities. Many demonstrate strong academic performance in subjects aligned with their cognitive strengths or special interests, while experiencing significant challenges with the social aspects of education. Assessment should explore this potential discrepancy, examining not only grades and test scores but also participation in group work, relationships with peers and teachers, and comfort in different educational environments.

Detailed educational history should examine patterns across different stages:

1. **Early education**: Initial adjustment to school environment, development of academic skills, early peer relationships, and response to classroom routines and expectations
2. **Primary education**: Academic strengths and challenges, friendship development, participation in various school activities, and beginning awareness of differences from peers

3. **Secondary education**: Response to increased social complexity, academic specialization, management of organizational demands, and preparation for post-secondary transitions
4. **Higher education (when applicable):** Course selection patterns, adjustment to independent learning, accommodation needs, social integration in university settings, and completion outcomes

This developmental perspective often reveals patterns of strength and challenge that reflect core autism features and their evolution over time.

Support received and accommodations needed throughout educational history can provide important information about both the nature of challenges and the types of support that have proven beneficial. Assessment should explore:

1. Formal academic accommodations received, such as extended time for assignments, alternative exam arrangements, or modified coursework
2. Informal supports provided by teachers, family members, or peers
3. Specific challenges that required accommodation, such as sensory sensitivities to classroom environments, difficulty with group projects, or executive functioning challenges affecting organization
4. Patterns of support needs across different educational contexts and developmental stages
5. Response to various types of educational intervention and support

Transitions between educational settings often represent particularly challenging periods for individuals with autism, highlighting difficulties with change, navigation of new social environments, and adaptation to different expectations and routines. Assessment should specifically explore experiences during transitions between:

1. Home or preschool to primary education
2. Primary to secondary education
3. Secondary to higher education or vocational training
4. Education to employment

Difficulties during these transition periods often provide important diagnostic information, as they reveal how the individual responds to disrupted routines, new social demands, and environments with different implicit expectations.

Employment history and current work functioning represent crucial domains for adult assessment, as occupational challenges are common even among individuals with strong cognitive and academic abilities:

Job acquisition and maintenance patterns may reveal autism-related challenges in areas such as:

1. Navigating the social aspects of job interviews
2. Adapting to changing job requirements or management
3. Understanding unwritten workplace rules and expectations
4. Managing executive functioning demands such as prioritization, time management, and multi-tasking
5. Sustaining employment despite strengths in job-specific skills

Assessment should explore the complete employment history, including reasons for job changes, patterns of success and challenge across different work environments, and the relationship between job requirements and individual strengths and challenges.

Workplace relationships often present significant challenges related to social communication differences. Assessment should examine:

1. Relationships with supervisors, including understanding of expectations, response to feedback, and communication patterns
2. Peer relationships with colleagues, including participation in workplace social activities, management of conflicts, and day-to-day social interactions
3. Customer or client interactions when relevant to the job role
4. Disclosure decisions regarding autism in workplace settings and the impact of disclosure or non-disclosure

Understanding these social dynamics provides important information about both the impact of autism on occupational functioning and potential areas for targeted support or accommodation.

Sensory aspects of work environments can significantly affect job performance and sustainability for many adults with autism. Assessment should explore:

1. Specific sensory challenges in current or past workplaces, such as noise levels, lighting, physical proximity to others, or other environmental factors
2. Accommodations that have been helpful in managing sensory challenges
3. Impact of sensory overload on work performance, attendance, and job retention
4. Strategies developed to manage sensory aspects of work environments

These sensory considerations often receive less attention than social or cognitive aspects of employment but may represent significant barriers to successful occupational functioning for many adults with autism.

Independent living skills assessment provides crucial information about day-to-day functioning and support needs:

Self-care and home management capabilities should be assessed comprehensively, including:

1. Personal hygiene and self-care routines
2. Meal planning, shopping, and preparation
3. Household cleaning and maintenance
4. Laundry and clothing care
5. Time management for daily activities
6. Adaptation to changes in routine or unexpected events

Assessment should consider not only whether the individual can perform these activities when prompted but whether they initiate and complete them independently and consistently. Many adults with autism can demonstrate skills in structured assessment situations that they struggle to implement consistently in daily life due to executive functioning challenges, motivation difficulties, or sensory barriers.

Financial management represents an area where many adults with autism experience challenges despite strong mathematical or technical abilities. Assessment should explore:

1. Budgeting and tracking expenses
2. Bill payment and account management
3. Understanding of financial concepts and requirements
4. Vulnerability to financial exploitation
5. Planning for future financial needs
6. Need for support or supervision with financial decisions

Executive functioning difficulties affecting planning, organization, and prospective memory may create significant challenges with financial management that are not immediately apparent from cognitive testing alone.

Transportation and community navigation involve multiple skills that may be affected by autism features, including:

1. Ability to use public transportation systems, including managing the sensory aspects of crowded transport and handling unexpected changes or delays
2. Driving skills and challenges, which may be affected by spatial processing, attention management, or anxiety
3. Wayfinding abilities in familiar and unfamiliar environments
4. Comfort and safety in community settings
5. Ability to access necessary community resources independently

These mobility and navigation skills significantly impact overall independence and community participation, making them important areas for functional assessment.

Relationships assessment examines the impact of autism features on various types of social connections:

Family dynamics may be significantly affected by autism features, with patterns that evolve over time. Assessment should explore:

1. Current relationships with family members, including parents, siblings, extended family, and children (if applicable)
2. Historical patterns in family relationships and how they have evolved with development and potential changes in understanding of autism
3. Family accommodation of autism features and its impact on family functioning
4. Communication patterns within the family system
5. Support provided by and to family members

Understanding family relationships provides important context for both diagnostic assessment and support planning, as families often represent crucial support systems for adults with autism.

Friendships should be assessed in terms of both quantity and quality:

1. Current friendship network and satisfaction with these relationships
2. Historical patterns in friendship development and maintenance
3. Types of activities shared with friends and contexts where friendships develop
4. Understanding of friendship concepts and expectations
5. Specific challenges in initiating and maintaining friendships
6. Strategies developed to navigate friendship relationships

Many adults with autism report significant challenges with friendship despite social interest, often describing confusion about friendship development, difficulty maintaining connections over time, or uncertainty about whether others consider them friends.

Intimate relationships present unique challenges that often become more apparent in adulthood:

1. History of romantic and sexual relationships
2. Current relationship status and satisfaction
3. Understanding of relationship expectations and dynamics
4. Communication patterns within intimate relationships
5. Management of sensory aspects of physical intimacy
6. Balancing relationship demands with need for solitude, routine, or special interest engagement

These intimate relationships often involve more complex social understanding, greater emotional reciprocity, and more nuanced communication than other relationship types, potentially creating challenges even for individuals who navigate other social contexts successfully.

Assessment tools for functional impact provide standardized approaches to evaluating adaptive functioning across domains:

The **World Health Organization Disability Assessment Schedule 2.0 (WHODAS 2.0)** offers a standardized approach to measuring health and disability across cultures. This 36-item instrument assesses functioning across six domains: cognition, mobility, self-care, getting along with others, life activities, and participation in society. It provides a global measure of functional impact that can be useful for documenting disability-related needs and measuring changes in functioning over time.

The **Vineland Adaptive Behaviour Scales, Third Edition (Vineland-3)** assesses adaptive behaviour across communication, daily living skills, socialization, and motor skills domains. While often associated with intellectual disability assessment, the Vineland-3 can provide valuable information about functional skills in autism without intellectual disability as well, particularly when there are questions about the gap between cognitive abilities and daily functioning.

The **Adaptive Behaviour Assessment System, Third Edition (ABAS-3)** provides another standardized measure of adaptive skills across conceptual, social, and practical domains. Like the Vineland-3, it offers both self-report and informant report versions, allowing comparison between self-perception and others' observations of functional skills.

Autism-specific functional measures include the **World Health Organization Quality of Life Assessment—Disabilities Module (WHOQOL-DIS),** which has been validated for use with adults with autism, and the **Functional Assessment Measure for Autism Spectrum Disorders (FAM-ASD),** which examines autism-specific functional challenges across multiple domains.

Integrating information from multiple sources is essential for accurate functional assessment, as individuals with autism may have limited insight into some functional challenges, while informants may lack awareness of the internal experience and effort associated with functioning. Combining self-report, informant report, direct observation, and historical information provides the most comprehensive understanding of functional impact.

The assessment of functional impact should ultimately aim not simply to document limitations but to identify specific barriers to optimal functioning that can be addressed through appropriate supports and accommodations. This strengths-based approach recognizes both challenges and capabilities, focusing on how environmental modifications, skill development, and targeted supports can enhance functioning and quality of life across domains.

CHAPTER 28

Formulation in ASD Assessment

Formulation represents a critical component of the autism assessment process, going beyond diagnosis to develop a comprehensive understanding of the individual's presentation that integrates assessment findings into a meaningful clinical narrative. While diagnosis addresses the categorical question of whether an individual meets criteria for autism spectrum disorder, formulation addresses the more complex questions of why this individual presents in this particular way, how various factors interact to create the current presentation, and what this understanding suggests for support and intervention. A sophisticated formulation integrates multiple theoretical perspectives, considers developmental trajectories and contextual factors, and provides the foundation for personalized support recommendations.

The purpose of formulation in autism assessment extends beyond simply justifying a diagnostic decision. Comprehensive formulation serves multiple functions:

1. It integrates diverse assessment information from various sources and measures into a coherent understanding of the individual's presentation
2. It explores the relationships between core autism features, co-occurring conditions, environmental factors, and adaptive responses
3. It provides a framework for understanding the development and maintenance of both challenges and strengths
4. It identifies potential targets for intervention and support
5. It offers a shared understanding that can be communicated to the individual, family members, and other professionals

When done effectively, formulation transforms a collection of assessment observations and scores into a meaningful narrative that enhances both understanding and intervention planning.

Components of comprehensive autism formulation include several key elements that should be addressed:

Core ASD features and their manifestation describes how the defining characteristics of autism—persistent differences in social communication and interaction, and restricted, repetitive patterns of behaviour, interests, or activities—present in this specific individual. This component should go beyond simply listing diagnostic criteria to explore the unique manifestation of autism features, including:

1. The specific nature of social communication differences, such as particular challenges with nonverbal communication, social reciprocity, or relationship development
2. The specific types of restricted and repetitive behaviour's present, such as special interests, sensory sensitivities, or need for sameness
3. The relative prominence of different autism features and their impact on functioning
4. How autism features manifest across different contexts and relationships

This detailed characterization of core features provides the foundation for understanding the individual's autism presentation and its functional implications.

Developmental trajectory and adaptations explore how autism features have evolved over time and how the individual has adapted to or compensated for challenges. This developmental perspective is essential for understanding the current presentation, as it reflects both neurodevelopmental differences and learned responses to those differences. Key aspects include:

1. Early developmental indicators of autism and their recognition or non-recognition
2. Changes in the manifestation of autism features across different developmental stages
3. Compensatory strategies developed to manage social, sensory, or executive functioning challenges
4. Impact of educational experiences, interventions, and support on developmental course
5. Critical periods or events that influenced development, such as transitions, losses, or significant successes

Understanding this developmental pathway helps explain why the individual presents as they do currently and provides context for both diagnosis and support planning.

Impact of environmental factors acknowledges that autism features do not exist in isolation but interact continuously with environmental demands, supports, and stressors. Formulation should consider:

1. How various environments (home, education, work, community) have accommodated or exacerbated autism-related challenges?
2. The impact of significant relationships on development and functioning
3. Cultural factors that have influenced the expression and interpretation of autism features
4. Socioeconomic factors affecting access to support, education, and intervention
5. Historical context, including changes in understanding and recognition of autism over the individual's lifetime

This ecological perspective recognizes that functioning reflects not only individual characteristics but the dynamic interaction between the person and their environment.

Comorbid conditions and their interactions address the complex relationships between autism and co-occurring physical, neurodevelopmental, and mental health conditions. Rather than viewing these as separate, distinct entities, formulation should explore:

1. Whether conditions developed as primary co-occurring conditions or secondary consequences of autism and associated experiences
2. How autism features may influence the presentation of other conditions (e.g., atypical presentation of anxiety or depression)
3. How other conditions may exacerbate or mask certain autism features
4. Potential shared neurobiological mechanisms underlying multiple conditions
5. The combined impact of autism and co-occurring conditions on functioning and quality of life

This integrated understanding of comorbidity is essential for effective intervention planning, as it guides decisions about which conditions to target and how to adapt interventions for the autism context.

Strengths and resources represent a crucial component that balances the clinical focus on challenges with recognition of capabilities, assets, and support systems. Comprehensive formulation should identify:

1. Cognitive and learning strengths that can be leveraged for skill development

2. Special interests that provide motivation, expertise, or potential vocational directions
3. Specific autism-related strengths such as attention to detail, pattern recognition, or logical analysis
4. Supportive relationships and environments that enhance functioning
5. Personal qualities such as determination, honesty, or creative thinking that represent resources for coping and development

This strengths-based perspective is essential for respectful, effective formulation that recognizes the whole person rather than focusing exclusively on difficulties.

Functional impact across domains examines how the interaction of all these factors affects the individual's participation and success in various life areas. This component connects clinical features to real-world outcomes, exploring:

1. How autism features, adaptations, environmental factors, comorbidities, and strengths collectively influence functioning in education, employment, relationships, independent living, and community participation
2. Specific barriers to optimal functioning in important life domains
3. Environmental modifications or supports that enhance functioning
4. The relationship between cognitive abilities and functional outcomes, particularly when there is a significant discrepancy
5. Subjective quality of life and satisfaction across domains

This functional analysis provides crucial information for prioritizing intervention targets and designing appropriate supports.

Several models provide theoretical frameworks for organizing and integrating these components into coherent formulation:

The **biopsychosocial model** offers a broad framework that considers biological factors (genetic predispositions, neurobiological differences), psychological processes (cognitive patterns, emotional responses, learning histories), and social contexts (relationships, cultural factors, socioeconomic circumstances). This integrated perspective is particularly valuable for autism formulation, as it avoids reductive biological explanations while acknowledging the neurobiological foundation of autism.

Developmental frameworks emphasize the dynamic nature of autism across the lifespan, considering how inherent neurodevelopmental differences interact with experience to shape developmental trajectories. These approaches recognize that development represents a continuous transaction between the individual and environment, with cascading effects of early differences on subsequent development. Developmental formulation explores how early autism features may have influenced learning opportunities, relationship development, and self-concept, creating pathways that explain current functioning.

Neurodiversity perspectives represent an important conceptual framework that views autism as a natural variation in human neurocognitive functioning rather than inherently a disorder or deficit. This approach acknowledges the genuine challenges associated with autism in neurotypically-designed environments while also recognizing the potential strengths and valuable cognitive differences that can accompany autism. Neurodiversity-informed formulation balances recognition of difficulties with respect for different ways of experiencing and interacting with the world.

The team approach to formulation brings together multiple professional perspectives to develop an integrated understanding that transcends disciplinary boundaries. This multidisciplinary integration is particularly valuable in autism assessment, as different team members bring complementary expertise:

1. Psychiatry contributes understanding of mental health comorbidities, neurobiological mechanisms, and potential pharmacological approaches
2. Psychology offers expertise in cognitive profiles, behavioural patterns, and psychological interventions
3. Speech and language therapy provides specialized assessment of communication strengths and challenges
4. Occupational therapy brings understanding of sensory processing, motor skills, and daily living capabilities
5. Education professionals contribute insights about learning styles and educational approaches
6. Social work perspectives highlight family dynamics, community resources, and socioeconomic factors

The most sophisticated formulations integrate these diverse perspectives into a cohesive understanding rather than presenting disconnected observations from different disciplines.

The process of developing comprehensive formulation typically involves several stages:

1. **Case discussion** brings together assessment information from multiple sources, with each team member contributing observations and interpretations from their disciplinary perspective. This initial sharing of information identifies patterns, discrepancies, and questions that require further exploration or integration.

2. **Collaborative formulation meetings** provide dedicated time for team members to develop an integrated understanding that transcends individual observations. These discussions move beyond reporting assessment findings to exploring the relationships between different aspects of the presentation and developing hypotheses about developmental pathways and maintaining factors.
3. **Formulation-focused supervision** offers opportunities to reflect on complex cases, consider alternative interpretations, and address potential biases or assumptions in the formulation process. This supervisory perspective can be particularly valuable when working with presentations that challenge typical understanding or require creative approaches to formulation.

Documentation of formulation should capture the richness of this integrative process while remaining accessible to both the individual being assessed and other professionals. Effective formulation documentation:

1. Provides a clear narrative that explains how the various assessment findings fit together
2. Uses language that is respectful and accessible while maintaining clinical precision
3. Balances recognition of challenges with acknowledgment of strengths and resources
4. Explicitly connects the formulation to recommendations for support and intervention
5. Acknowledges areas of uncertainty or alternative interpretations when appropriate

Well-documented formulation serves as a valuable reference for future support planning and helps ensure continuity of understanding across different professionals and services.

The ultimate goal of formulation in autism assessment is to develop an understanding that is not only clinically sophisticated but also meaningful and useful to the individual and those who support them. Effective formulation enhances self-understanding, guides intervention planning, and provides a framework for making sense of past experiences and navigating future challenges. By moving beyond diagnosis to comprehensive formulation, clinicians provide a foundation for truly personalized, effective support that recognizes and responds to the unique constellation of factors that shape each individual's autism presentation.

CHAPTER 29

Diagnostic Decision Making

Diagnostic decision making in adult autism assessment represents the culmination of a complex clinical process that integrates multiple sources of information to reach conclusions about whether an individual meets criteria for autism spectrum disorder. This process requires sophisticated clinical judgment, careful consideration of diagnostic criteria, awareness of potential biases, and thoughtful management of diagnostic uncertainty. Understanding the principles and challenges of diagnostic decision making is essential for consistent, accurate, and ethical diagnostic practice.

ICD-11 criteria serve as the primary diagnostic framework for UK clinical practice. The current **International Classification of Diseases (11th edition)** defines autism spectrum disorder (code 6A02) as characterized by:

1. Persistent deficits in the ability to initiate and sustain reciprocal social interaction and social communication
2. A range of restricted, repetitive, and inflexible patterns of behaviour, interests, or activities
3. Onset during the developmental period, typically early childhood, though symptoms may not become fully manifest until later
4. Symptoms cause clinically significant impairment in personal, family, social, educational, occupational, or other important areas of functioning

The ICD-11 framework includes several important specifiers that provide additional information about the individual's presentation:

- **6A02.0** Autism Spectrum Disorder without disorder of intellectual development and with mild or no impairment of functional language
- **6A02.1** Autism Spectrum Disorder with disorder of intellectual development and with mild or no impairment of functional language
- **6A02.2** Autism Spectrum Disorder without disorder of intellectual development and with impaired functional language

- **6A02.3** Autism Spectrum Disorder with disorder of intellectual development and with impaired functional language
- **6A02.4** Autism Spectrum Disorder without disorder of intellectual development and with absence of functional language
- **6A02.5** Autism Spectrum Disorder with disorder of intellectual development and with absence of functional language
- **6A02.Y** Other specified Autism Spectrum Disorder
- **6A02.Z** Autism Spectrum Disorder, unspecified

These specifiers for intellectual functioning and functional language provide valuable clinical information about the presentation and likely support needs, moving beyond a simple binary diagnosis to a more nuanced classification. When applying these specifiers, "disorder of intellectual development" refers to intellectual functioning significantly below the average range (generally IQ < 70), while functional language refers to the individual's ability to use language for functional communication rather than simply the presence of speech.

The dimensional approach to autism diagnosis has evolved significantly in recent diagnostic systems, reflecting growing recognition that autism features exist on continua rather than as categorical distinctions. This dimensional conceptualization acknowledges variation in:

1. Severity of social communication difficulties
2. Severity of restricted and repetitive behaviour patterns
3. Intellectual functioning
4. Language abilities
5. Functional impact across domains

Rather than focusing solely on whether an individual meets diagnostic threshold, this approach considers the specific pattern and intensity of autism features across multiple dimensions. This more nuanced understanding supports individualized assessment and intervention planning while acknowledging the heterogeneity within autism.

Severity levels can be specified across different domains of functioning, though ICD-11 does not mandate a specific severity rating system (unlike DSM-5, which includes three severity levels). Clinical practice in the UK often involves describing the degree of support needed across different functional domains rather than assigning global severity ratings. This approach recognizes that individuals may require different levels of support across different areas of functioning—for example, minimal support for daily living skills but substantial support for workplace social interaction.

Confidence levels in diagnostic decisions should be explicitly considered and communicated, particularly in complex or borderline cases. Rather than presenting all diagnostic conclusions with equal certainty, clinicians should indicate the degree of confidence in the diagnosis using terminology such as:

Definite: Strong evidence across multiple sources clearly supports diagnosis, with minimal contradictory information and good agreement among team members **Probable:** Preponderance of evidence supports diagnosis, though some features may be less clear or some sources may provide contradictory information Possible: Some evidence supports diagnosis, but significant uncertainty remains due to limited information, conflicting evidence, or alternative explanations

This transparent approach to diagnostic confidence acknowledges the inherent uncertainty in some clinical presentations and supports appropriate caution in diagnostic conclusions when warranted.

Consensus process within multidisciplinary teams represents best practice for diagnostic decision making in adult autism assessment. Rather than relying on a single clinician's judgment, team-based approaches bring together multiple professional perspectives and areas of expertise to reach diagnostic conclusions. This consensus process typically involves:

1. Independent formulation of initial impressions by different team members based on their assessment components
2. Structured team discussion of assessment findings across domains
3. Explicit consideration of how the evidence aligns with diagnostic criteria
4. Exploration of alternative explanations for the presenting difficulties
5. Resolution of discrepancies between different sources of information
6. Reaching consensus on diagnostic conclusions and confidence levels

This collaborative approach enhances diagnostic accuracy, reduces individual bias, and ensures that diverse perspectives inform the diagnostic decision. When team members disagree, thorough discussion of the reasons for differing interpretations often leads to a more nuanced understanding of the presentation.

Diagnostic uncertainty requires thoughtful management in clinical practice. When there is insufficient information for definitive diagnosis, several approaches may be appropriate:

1. Extended assessment period: Additional assessment sessions, observations in different contexts, or collection of further collateral information may resolve uncertainty

2. Trial interventions: Implementing autism-specific supports and monitoring response can sometimes provide additional diagnostic information
3. Developmental monitoring: For younger adults, observing developmental progression over time may clarify diagnostic questions
4. Second opinion: Referral to clinicians with specialized expertise in complex or atypical presentations may be appropriate in cases of significant uncertainty

When uncertainty persists despite thorough assessment, transparent communication about the limits of diagnostic certainty is essential. Provisional diagnoses with plans for review, descriptions of the individual's profile without definitive categorical diagnosis, or explicit acknowledgment of features consistent with autism alongside other conditions may be appropriate in such cases.

Documentation of diagnostic decisions should include not only the conclusion but the reasoning process that led to it. Effective diagnostic documentation includes:

1. Explicit reference to how the individual's presentation meets specific diagnostic criteria
2. Discussion of the pattern of evidence across different assessment components
3. Consideration of alternative explanations and why they were ruled out
4. Acknowledgment of any contradictory or inconsistent information
5. Clear statement of diagnostic confidence and any remaining uncertainty
6. Explanation of any specifiers applied and their clinical significance

This transparent documentation supports consistent understanding across professionals, clarifies the basis for diagnostic conclusions, and provides a foundation for future reassessment if needed.

Cultural considerations significantly impact diagnostic decision making and require explicit attention throughout the assessment process. Cultural factors influence:

1. The interpretation of social communication patterns, as norms for eye contact, conversational style, emotional expression, and social relationships vary considerably across cultures
2. The identification of restricted or repetitive behaviours, as what constitutes unusual interests or excessive adherence to routines may differ across cultural contexts
3. The reporting and interpretation of developmental history, as milestones and expectations vary culturally

4. The perceived impact of behavioural differences, as functional expectations differ across cultures
5. The acceptability and understanding of diagnostic labels, which have different meanings and implications across cultural contexts

Culturally informed diagnostic decision making requires recognition of these influences, adaptation of interpretation frameworks to the individual's cultural context, and involvement of cultural consultants when assessing individuals from cultural backgrounds different from the clinician's own experience.

Several potential biases can influence diagnostic decision making and should be consciously addressed:

1. Confirmation bias leads clinicians to notice and emphasize information that confirms initial impressions while minimizing contradictory evidence. This can be mitigated by explicitly seeking disconfirming information and considering alternative explanations.
2. Anchoring bias involves giving too much weight to initial information or impressions, such as referral information or presenting complaints. Using structured assessment protocols and deliberately considering all evidence before forming conclusions helps counter this tendency.
3. Availability bias leads to overemphasis on familiar or recently encountered presentations. Regular clinical supervision, team-based decision making, and reference to current research and diagnostic criteria help maintain balanced clinical judgment.
4. Gender bias has historically contributed to underdiagnosis of autism in females. Awareness of gender differences in autism presentation, use of gender-sensitive assessment approaches, and critical examination of assumptions about "typical" autism presentations are essential for equitable diagnostic practice.
5. Diagnostic overshadowing involves attributing all difficulties to a primary diagnosis without recognizing co-occurring conditions. Comprehensive assessment that systematically explores potential comorbidities helps prevent this oversimplification.

Conscious awareness of these potential biases, combined with structured assessment approaches, team-based decision making, and regular reflective practice, supports more accurate and consistent diagnostic conclusions.

The ultimate purpose of diagnostic decision making extends beyond categorization to providing a foundation for understanding and support. Diagnosis should serve as a tool for accessing appropriate services, developing effective interventions, enhancing self-understanding, and connecting with relevant communities. This purpose-oriented approach maintains focus on how diagnostic decisions can benefit the individual rather than diagnosis as an end in itself.

By combining rigorous application of diagnostic criteria with clinical wisdom, cultural sensitivity, and transparent management of uncertainty, clinicians can make diagnostic decisions that are both scientifically sound and clinically meaningful, providing a solid foundation for subsequent support and intervention planning.

CHAPTER 30
Writing the Diagnostic Report

The diagnostic report represents the formal documentation of the autism assessment process, findings, and conclusions. As the enduring record of the assessment, this document serves multiple important functions: it communicates assessment findings to the individual and referrer, provides justification for diagnostic decisions, establishes a foundation for support planning, and serves as a reference for future providers. A well-crafted diagnostic report balances comprehensive clinical detail with accessibility, provides meaningful interpretation of assessment findings, and translates clinical conclusions into practical recommendations. Understanding the principles of effective report writing is essential for creating documents that serve both clinical and practical purposes.

The structure of a comprehensive autism diagnostic report typically includes several key sections, each serving specific functions in documenting the assessment process and findings:

Referral information establishes the context for the assessment, including:

1. Source of referral and date received
2. Reason for referral, including specific questions or concerns
3. Background information provided with the referral
4. Previous assessments or diagnoses relevant to the current evaluation

This section documents why the assessment was conducted and what specific questions it aimed to address, providing important context for the subsequent findings and conclusions.

Assessment methods detail the specific approaches used to gather information, including:

1. Direct assessment sessions: dates, duration, and content
2. Standardized instruments administered, with version numbers and dates of administration

3. Informant interviews: who was interviewed, when, and what information was sought
4. Documents reviewed, such as educational or medical records
5. Observations in different contexts, if applicable

This methodological transparency documents the comprehensiveness of the assessment approach and allows readers to evaluate the strength of the evidence base for diagnostic conclusions.

Developmental history summarizes key information about early development and its progression, including:

1. Pregnancy, birth, and early milestone development
2. Early social communication development
3. Language acquisition and development
4. Play and peer interaction in early childhood
5. Educational history and adjustments
6. Previous interventions or supports and their impact
7. Developmental trajectory across different domains

This historical perspective is essential for establishing the developmental nature of autism and understanding how features have manifested and evolved over time.

Current presentation describes findings from direct assessment and collateral information about current functioning, organized by relevant domains:

1. Social communication and interaction:
    - Nonverbal communication (eye contact, facial expression, gesture)
    - Reciprocal conversation and social reciprocity
    - Relationship development and maintenance
    - Social understanding and perspective-taking
2. Restricted and repetitive behaviours:
    - Special interests: content, intensity, and social sharing
    - Routines, rituals, and response to change
    - Repetitive movements and behaviours
    - Sensory sensitivities and interests
3. Associated features:
    - Cognitive and language abilities

- Executive functioning
- Emotional regulation
- Adaptive functioning across domains

This detailed description of current functioning provides the primary evidence base for diagnostic conclusions and identifies specific strengths and challenges that inform support recommendations.

Standardized assessment results present findings from formal assessment measures, including:

1. Names of instruments and dates administered
2. Scores and classifications, with reference to normative expectations
3. Qualitative observations during standardized assessment
4. Integration of findings across different measures
5. Limitations or contextual factors affecting interpretation of results

This objective documentation of standardized assessment findings provides empirical support for clinical impressions and allows comparison to established norms and criteria.

Formulation integrates assessment information into a meaningful understanding of the individual's presentation, addressing:

1. How various assessment findings fit together to create a coherent clinical picture
2. Developmental pathways that explain the current presentation
3. Interaction between autism features, co-occurring conditions, and environmental factors
4. Strengths and resources alongside challenges
5. Factors that have helped or hindered development and adaptation

This interpretive section moves beyond description to explanation, helping the individual and others understand not just what has been observed but why the person presents as they do.

Diagnosis and diagnostic reasoning present conclusions about diagnosis with explicit rationale:

1. Clear statement of diagnostic conclusions, including any specifiers
2. Explicit reference to how the presentation meets specific diagnostic criteria
3. Discussion of diagnostic confidence and any areas of uncertainty
4. Consideration of alternative explanations and differential diagnosis

5. Explanation of any co-occurring conditions identified

This transparent reasoning process documents the basis for diagnostic decisions and helps others understand the clinical judgment applied in reaching conclusions.

Recommendations provides specific guidance for support and intervention based on assessment findings:

1. Educational or occupational accommodations and supports
2. Psychological or therapeutic interventions for identified needs
3. Environmental adaptations to address sensory or executive functioning challenges
4. Approaches for developing specific skills or managing difficulties
5. Resources, services, or benefits for which the individual may be eligible
6. Suggestions for family members, partners, or employers on supporting the individual

This action-oriented section translates assessment findings into practical next steps, ensuring the assessment leads to meaningful support.

Language Considerations in Diagnostic Reporting

Language considerations significantly impact the accessibility and usefulness of diagnostic reports. Effective reports balance professional terminology with clear, straightforward expression that can be understood by non-specialists. Key principles include:

Clear, specific language that avoids ambiguity and vague generalizations in favour of precise description. Rather than stating that someone "has poor social skills," effective reports specify exactly what was observed: "struggles to maintain reciprocal conversation, with a tendency to shift topics abruptly to personal interests without recognizing the conversation partner's cues of disinterest." This specificity provides much more useful information for understanding and support planning.

Technical terminology should be used judiciously and always explained when introduced. When specialized terms are necessary for precision or to facilitate communication with other professionals, they should be accompanied by plain language explanations: "demonstrated significant pragmatic language difficulties (problems using language appropriately in social contexts), specifically struggling to adapt communication style to different listeners and situations."

Accessible structure that enhances comprehension through logical organization, clear headings, appropriate paragraph breaks, and judicious use of bullet points for complex information. Visual formatting that distinguishes between different types of information helps readers navigate the document and locate specific content.

Reports should be written at an appropriate reading level for the intended audience, typically aiming for secondary school level (around 9th-10th grade in the US system) to ensure accessibility while maintaining necessary content. Sentence length, vocabulary complexity, and explanation of concepts should be calibrated to this reading level.

Strengths-based language represents an important ethical consideration in report writing. While diagnostic reports must document difficulties to justify diagnosis and identify support needs, they should also:

Highlight abilities alongside challenges, providing a balanced view of the individual rather than focusing exclusively on deficits. This balanced approach more accurately represents the person's complete profile and helps identify strengths that can be leveraged in intervention planning.

Use respectful language that describes behaviours and experiences without pejorative judgment. For example, rather than describing someone as "failing to make eye contact," the report might state that the person "makes limited eye contact during conversation, typically looking at objects or to the side rather than at the conversation partner's face."

Frame differences in neutral terms rather than inherently pathologizing language. For instance, describing "differences in social approach" rather than "abnormal social behaviour" acknowledges the different neurodevelopmental trajectory without unnecessarily negative connotations.

Respect the individual's identity and preferences regarding terminology, particularly in relation to identity-first language ("autistic person") versus person-first language ("person with autism"). When the individual has expressed a clear preference, this should be respected throughout the report.

This strengths-based approach does not minimize challenges or avoid clear diagnostic language but ensures that the report presents a respectful, holistic view of the individual that supports dignity and self-esteem alongside accurate clinical documentation.

Purpose of the report should always guide decisions about content, structure, and language. Diagnostic reports typically serve multiple audiences and purposes, including:

Document for the patient that explains their diagnosis, validates their experiences, enhances self-understanding, and provides a foundation for self-advocacy. This purpose requires accessible language, clear explanations of technical concepts, and explicit connections between diagnostic findings and lived experience.

Record for the referrer that answers the referral questions, justifies diagnostic conclusions, and provides guidance for next steps. This purpose requires clear diagnostic statements, explicit reasoning, and specific, actionable recommendations.

Reference for future providers that documents the assessment process, findings, and conclusions to inform future care. This purpose requires comprehensive documentation of methods and results, including technical details that may be relevant to other clinicians.

Official document for services and benefits that establishes eligibility for support. This purpose requires explicit statements about diagnosis and functional impact that align with eligibility criteria for relevant services and accommodations.

Balancing these different purposes requires thoughtful decisions about what to include, how to structure information, and what language to use. In some cases, providing separate documents for different audiences (such as a technical report for other clinicians and an accessible summary for the individual) may best serve these varied purposes.

UK requirements for NHS report standards and information governance place additional parameters on diagnostic report writing. These include:

- Compliance with NHS Digital Record Keeping Standards, which specify requirements for accuracy, comprehensiveness, contemporaneousness, and security of clinical documentation
- Adherence to information governance principles regarding confidentiality, data protection, and appropriate sharing of information
- Inclusion of specific administrative elements such as NHS number, demographic information, and service identifiers
- Clear documentation of consent for assessment and for information sharing
- Appropriate clinical coding using current ICD-11 classifications
- Compliance with local trust or service requirements for report format and content

These formal requirements ensure that diagnostic reports meet professional and legal standards while serving their clinical and practical purposes.

The writing process for high-quality diagnostic reports typically involves several stages:

1. Immediate post-assessment documentation of observations and findings, when details are fresh in the clinician's mind
2. Team discussion and formulation to integrate findings across different assessment components
3. Drafting the report with reference to notes, assessment results, and team formulation
4. Review and editing for clarity, completeness, and appropriate language
5. Team review in complex or challenging cases to ensure accuracy and comprehensiveness
6. Final formatting and preparation for sharing with the individual and, with consent, other relevant parties

This structured process ensures that reports accurately reflect the assessment findings, integrate multiple perspectives, and communicate effectively with their intended audiences.

Quality assurance for diagnostic reports may include peer review processes, supervision of report writing for less experienced clinicians, use of report templates or frameworks to ensure consistency, and periodic audit of reports against quality standards. These processes help maintain high standards of report writing across services and clinicians.

CHAPTER 31
Feedback Session

The feedback session represents a critical component of the autism assessment process, providing the opportunity to share diagnostic conclusions, explain assessment findings, and discuss their implications with the individual being assessed. Far more than simply communicating a diagnostic label, this session serves multiple important purposes: it helps the person understand the meaning of the diagnosis in the context of their life experiences, validates their lived experience, provides a foundation for identity development and self-advocacy, and establishes a direction for future support. When conducted with skill and sensitivity, the feedback session can be a transformative experience that initiates a positive process of self-understanding and adaptation.

Preparation for the feedback session is essential to ensure that this important conversation proceeds effectively. Key preparatory elements include:

Anticipating emotional responses that allows the clinician to prepare for the range of reactions that individuals may have to receiving an autism diagnosis. These reactions vary widely and may include:

1. **Relief and validation**: Many adults report that diagnosis provides a framework for understanding lifelong difficulties and differences, validating experiences that may previously have been attributed to personal failings
2. **Grief or loss:** Some individuals experience grief related to late identification, missed opportunities, or adjustment to a new understanding of themselves
3. **Shock or disbelief**: Despite seeking assessment, some people may be surprised by a positive diagnosis, particularly if they have internalized different explanations for their experiences
4. **Anxiety about the future**: Concerns about what the diagnosis means for relationships, employment, or independence
5. **Anger about missed earlier identification**: Feelings of frustration or resentment about previous misdiagnoses or lack of support

6. **Confusion about what the diagnosis means**: Uncertainty about how autism affects them specifically or what happens next

Preparing for these varied reactions involves planning sufficient time for the session, ensuring a comfortable and private environment, considering who should be present to provide support, and developing approaches for addressing different emotional responses compassionately and effectively.

Accessible explanation materials support understanding of complex assessment information. These might include:

1. Visual aids such as diagrams illustrating autism features or spectrum concepts
2. Written summaries of key assessment findings and their meaning
3. Simplified explanations of diagnostic criteria and how they apply to the individual
4. Case examples or scenarios that illustrate autism features in everyday life
5. Analogies or metaphors that help explain neurodevelopmental differences
6. Information about autism written by autistic individuals that provides lived experience perspectives

Having these materials prepared in advance allows the clinician to select appropriate resources based on the individual's information processing style, cognitive profile, and specific questions or concerns.

Supporting the person's preferences for how feedback is provided demonstrates respect for their autonomy and enhances the effectiveness of communication. Considerations include:

1. Written summary provided before or during the session for those who process written information more effectively than verbal
2. Visual aids for those who think visually or benefit from visual structure
3. Presence or absence of support persons based on the individual's comfort with discussing personal information
4. Pacing of information delivery based on processing speed and emotional readiness
5. Balance between technical precision and accessible language based on the individual's background knowledge and preferences
6. Options for follow-up questions after the initial feedback, recognizing that processing complex information may take time

When possible, discussing these preferences before the feedback session allows for tailored preparation that respects the individual's communication and processing needs.

The structure of the feedback session should provide a coherent framework for sharing complex information while remaining flexible enough to respond to the individual's reactions and questions. An effective structure typically includes:

Review of the assessment process helps orient the individual to what has been done and why, establishing context for the findings about to be shared. This review might include:

1. Reminder of the referral questions or reasons for seeking assessment
2. Summary of assessment components completed (interviews, standardized measures, observations)
3. Information gathered from different sources (self-report, informant report, records)
4. Acknowledgment of the individual's participation and contribution to the process

This orientation helps the person understand the comprehensive nature of the assessment and the solid foundation for the conclusions that will be discussed.

Explanation of findings should present assessment results in a clear, organized manner that helps the individual understand both the evidence for diagnosis and the specific nature of their autism presentation. This explanation typically addresses:

1. Patterns observed across different assessment components
2. Specific autism features identified and how they manifest in this individual
3. Strengths and abilities alongside challenges
4. How assessment findings connect to the person's reported experiences and concerns
5. Results of standardized measures in accessible language
6. Integration of different perspectives (self, informant, clinician observations)

This detailed explanation provides the evidential basis for diagnostic conclusions while helping the person understand their unique profile rather than just a diagnostic category.

Diagnosis and what it means involves clear communication of diagnostic conclusions with explanation of their significance. This discussion includes:

1. Explicit statement of diagnostic conclusions, including any specifiers

2. Explanation of what autism means as a neurodevelopmental condition
3. Discussion of how autism manifests specifically in this individual
4. Clarification of what the diagnosis does not mean (addressing common misconceptions)
5. Explanation of any diagnostic uncertainty or limitations in the assessment
6. Discussion of any co-occurring conditions identified and their relationship to autism

This component translates clinical conclusions into meaningful understanding, helping the person integrate the diagnosis into their self-concept in an accurate and constructive way.

Strength identification represents a crucial component that balances discussion of challenges with recognition of positive qualities and abilities. This includes:

1. Cognitive and learning strengths identified during assessment
2. Personal qualities that represent resources for coping and development
3. Specific autism-related strengths such as attention to detail, pattern recognition, or perseverance
4. Skills and competencies developed despite challenges
5. Interests and passions that provide motivation and potential growth directions

This strengths-based discussion helps counter potential negative impacts of diagnosis by emphasizing capabilities and resources alongside support needs.

Impact on daily life connects abstract diagnostic concepts to concrete lived experience, helping the person understand how autism affects their day-to-day functioning. This discussion explores:

1. How identified autism features influence specific life domains such as education, employment, relationships, and independent living
2. Explanation of past experiences or challenges through the lens of autism
3. Understanding of specific difficulties that have prompted concern or help-seeking
4. Recognition of adaptations or compensatory strategies already developed
5. Identification of specific barriers to optimal functioning that might be addressed through support

This practical application of diagnostic understanding helps the person recognize the relevance of the diagnosis to their life circumstances and challenges.

Recommendations and next steps translate assessment findings into constructive action, providing direction for moving forward after diagnosis. This discussion covers:

1. Specific recommendations for support, intervention, or accommodation
2. Resources for learning more about autism (books, websites, organizations)
3. Options for post-diagnostic support services
4. Information about benefits, accommodations, or services for which the diagnosis may establish eligibility
5. Suggestions for sharing diagnostic information with others (family, employers, educators) if desired
6. Plan for any follow-up appointments or referrals

This future-oriented component ensures that diagnosis leads to practical benefit rather than simply providing a label without direction for support.

Supporting understanding during the feedback session requires specific skills and approaches that help the person process complex information about themselves:

Check comprehension regularly throughout the session, using approaches such as:

1. Asking the person to summarize their understanding of key points
2. Inviting questions at natural breaks in the discussion
3. Watching for nonverbal cues of confusion or misunderstanding
4. Offering alternative explanations when initial explanations don't seem to connect
5. Checking emotional reactions as well as cognitive understanding

This active monitoring of comprehension allows for clarification of misunderstandings and adaptation of communication to enhance understanding.

Space for questions should be explicitly provided and supported, recognizing that:

1. Processing complex personal information takes time, and questions may emerge gradually
2. Some individuals may need encouragement to ask questions, particularly if they have difficulty formulating questions in the moment
3. Written questions prepared in advance may be easier for some people than spontaneous verbal questions
4. Some questions may reflect concerns about implications rather than requests for information

5. Questions may continue to arise after the initial feedback session as the person processes the diagnosis

Creating a supportive atmosphere for questions involves explicitly inviting them, responding without judgment, acknowledging good questions, and providing multiple opportunities and modalities for asking questions both during and after the feedback session.

Written materials to take home provide ongoing reference after the initial feedback, supporting continued processing and understanding. These materials might include:

1. A draft or summary of the diagnostic report
2. Handouts explaining autism in general and how it relates to the individual specifically
3. Lists of recommended resources for further learning
4. Written explanations of recommendations and next steps
5. Contact information for follow-up questions or concerns
6. Information about local support services and how to access them

These take-home materials recognize that processing diagnosis is an ongoing process rather than a one-time event, providing resources that support this extended integration of diagnostic understanding.

Involving support persons in the feedback session can provide emotional support and enhance understanding but should be approached with careful consideration of the individual's preferences and needs. Key considerations include:

With consent from the individual being assessed, support persons such as partners, family members, or close friends may be included in all or part of the feedback session. Their presence can:

1. Provide emotional support during a potentially overwhelming experience
2. Help remember and process complex information
3. Develop shared understanding that supports ongoing adaptation
4. Ask questions the individual might not think to ask
5. Begin to understand how they can best support the person

However, the presence of others may also inhibit the individual's honest reaction or questions, particularly if there are relationship tensions or if the support person has their own strong emotional responses to the diagnosis. The decision about including others should prioritize the needs and preferences of the person being assessed while recognizing the potential value of shared understanding.

For some adults, particularly those with significant anxiety, communication differences, or difficulties processing verbal information, having a trusted support person present may be essential for effective feedback. In these cases, preparation with both the individual and their support person can help ensure that the support person's presence enhances rather than impedes the feedback process.

Following the feedback session, providing opportunities for additional questions or clarification acknowledges that processing diagnostic information takes time and that understanding evolves with reflection. Options for follow-up might include:

1. A scheduled follow-up appointment specifically for questions that arise after initial feedback
2. Telephone or email contact for brief clarifications
3. Referral to post-diagnostic support groups where questions can be explored with peers and professionals
4. Provision of resources that address common questions following diagnosis

This extended support for processing diagnostic information recognizes diagnosis as the beginning of a journey of understanding rather than a conclusive endpoint.

CHAPTER 32
Diagnostic Uncertainty

While many autisms assessments lead to clear diagnostic conclusions, clinicians regularly encounter cases where diagnostic certainty is more elusive. These situations of diagnostic uncertainty require specific approaches to assessment, formulation, and communication that maintain clinical integrity while acknowledging the limitations of current diagnostic frameworks. Understanding how to manage diagnostic uncertainty is an essential skill for all clinicians involved in autism assessment, allowing for appropriate caution in complex cases while still providing helpful formulation and support recommendations.

Several common reasons for uncertainty in adult autism assessment arise from various limitations in the assessment process, the diagnostic criteria, or the presentation itself:

Incomplete developmental information frequently complicates adult assessment, particularly for older adults whose parents may be deceased or unavailable, or when childhood records have been lost or destroyed. Without reliable information about early development, determining whether current features represent lifelong neurodevelopmental differences or later-acquired patterns becomes more challenging. This limitation can be particularly significant when assessing individuals who may have had subtle presentations in childhood that became more apparent with increasing social demands in adolescence or adulthood.

Masked presentation due to effective compensatory strategies can create significant diagnostic uncertainty. Many adults, particularly those with higher cognitive abilities, develop sophisticated approaches to managing social communication challenges and concealing repetitive behaviours or sensory sensitivities in assessment settings. These compensatory strategies may be so effective that autism features become apparent only in situations of high stress, novel demands, or when compensation breaks down due to exhaustion or mental health challenges. Identifying these masked presentations requires careful assessment across multiple contexts and detailed exploration of the subjective experience of social interaction, including the effort required and aftermath experienced.

Complex comorbidities can obscure the diagnostic picture when multiple conditions with overlapping features co-occur. For example, social withdrawal and restricted interests might reflect autism, social anxiety disorder, obsessive-compulsive disorder, or some combination of these conditions. Untangling these complex presentations requires careful exploration of the developmental trajectory of different symptoms, their underlying mechanisms, and their relationship to each other. This complexity often necessitates extended assessment over multiple sessions and input from clinicians with expertise in various conditions.

Borderline presentations that partially meet diagnostic criteria but fall short of full clinical threshold create particular challenges for categorical diagnostic systems. These sub-threshold presentations may nonetheless cause significant functional impairment and benefit from autism-informed support approaches. The dimensional nature of autism features means that some individuals will inevitably fall at the boundaries of current diagnostic categories, requiring careful clinical judgment about whether diagnosis is appropriate and helpful.

Management approaches for cases with diagnostic uncertainty should balance appropriate clinical caution with practical support for the individual's needs:

Extended assessment period may be warranted when initial evaluation yields inconclusive findings. This extended approach might include:

1. Additional assessment sessions in different contexts or settings
2. Observation in naturalistic environments such as workplace or educational settings
3. More extensive collection of collateral information from multiple sources
4. Assessment during periods of higher stress when compensation may be less effective
5. Reassessment after significant life transitions that might reveal underlying differences

This extended approach recognizes that some presentations require more comprehensive assessment than can be accomplished in a standard assessment protocol, particularly when features are subtle or masked.

Trial interventions can sometimes provide valuable diagnostic information when standard assessment yields uncertainty. Implementing autism-specific supports and monitoring response may clarify whether the individual's difficulties align with an autism profile. For example:

1. Environmental modifications addressing sensory sensitivities
2. Explicit teaching of social communication strategies
3. Support for executive functioning challenges using autism-informed approaches
4. Structured approaches to managing change and transitions

Positive response to these autism-specific interventions provides supportive evidence for diagnosis, while limited response might suggest alternative explanations for the presenting difficulties. However, this approach should be used cautiously and never as the sole basis for diagnostic decisions, as response to intervention is influenced by many factors beyond diagnostic classification.

Developmental monitoring over time may be appropriate for younger adults with unclear presentations, allowing observation of how features evolve with further development and changing life demands. This longitudinal perspective can be particularly valuable for individuals in transition periods such as:

1. Moving from education to employment
2. Leaving the family home for independent living
3. Developing more complex intimate relationships
4. Taking on new roles with increased social or executive functioning demands

These transitions often reveal previously masked difficulties or clarify the nature of existing challenges, providing additional information for diagnostic decision-making.

Second opinion from clinicians with specialized expertise may be warranted in particularly complex or challenging cases. Referral for second opinion might be considered when:

1. The presentation includes unusual or atypical features
2. Standard assessment approaches yield contradictory information
3. The clinical team has limited experience with similar presentations
4. There are significant disagreements within the assessment team about diagnosis
5. The individual or family has strong concerns about the initial assessment conclusions

This approach acknowledges the limitations of individual clinical judgment and leverages specialized expertise for particularly challenging cases.

Documentation of diagnostic uncertainty requires transparent communication in clinical records and reports. This documentation should include:

Clearly stating degree of certainty using explicit language about confidence levels, such as "possible," "probable," or "definite" autism, or by describing the presentation as "having features consistent with autism spectrum disorder" rather than making a definitive diagnosis when uncertainty is significant.

Explaining specific reasons for uncertainty helps others understand the nature of the diagnostic challenges and the basis for clinical caution. This explanation might address:

1. Specific missing information that would clarify diagnosis if available
2. Contradictory findings across different assessment components
3. Features that align with autism alongside features that suggest alternative explanations
4. Contextual factors that complicate interpretation of assessment findings
5. Developmental or historical factors that remain unclear

This transparency about the reasons for uncertainty helps the individual and others understand the nature of the diagnostic complexity rather than perceiving uncertainty as clinical indecisiveness.

Describing features consistent with autism while acknowledging diagnostic limitations allows for useful clinical formulation despite uncertainty. This approach might involve:

1. Detailing specific social communication differences observed, regardless of whether they reach diagnostic threshold
2. Describing restricted and repetitive behaviour patterns and their impact on functioning
3. Explaining how these features relate to the individual's presenting concerns
4. Acknowledging limitations in determining whether these features reflect autism or alternative explanations

This feature-focused approach provides useful clinical understanding while maintaining appropriate caution about diagnostic classification.

Formulating alternative explanations that might account for the presenting difficulties demonstrates thoroughness and diagnostic rigor. This might include:

1. Other neurodevelopmental conditions that share features with autism

2. Mental health conditions that might explain some or all of the observed features
3. Personality factors or traits that might account for social or behavioural patterns
4. Environmental or contextual factors that might contribute to current functioning

Explicitly considering these alternatives shows that diagnostic uncertainty reflects careful consideration of multiple explanations rather than inadequate assessment.

Communication with the individual about diagnostic uncertainty requires particular skill and sensitivity. Key principles include:

Transparent discussion of the assessment findings and their implications, avoiding both false certainty and unnecessarily vague conclusions. This involves:

1. Clear explanation of what is known based on the assessment
2. Honest acknowledgment of what remains uncertain
3. Explanation of the reasons for uncertainty in accessible language
4. Discussion of the limitations of current diagnostic frameworks
5. Exploration of what diagnostic information means for the individual, regardless of certainty

This transparent approach respects the individual's right to understand their assessment results while maintaining clinical integrity in acknowledging limitations.

Focusing on formulation rather than diagnostic classification can provide meaningful understanding despite uncertainty. This approach emphasizes:

1. The pattern of strengths and challenges identified, regardless of diagnostic label
2. How these patterns help explain the individual's experiences and difficulties
3. Factors that influence functioning positively and negatively
4. Approaches that might be helpful based on the identified patterns

This formulation-focused communication provides useful understanding without requiring definitive diagnostic conclusions.

Discussing implications for support emphasizes practical benefit over diagnostic certainty. This discussion addresses:

1. Specific support approaches that might be helpful based on identified needs
2. How understanding of the individual's profile can inform adaptations and accommodations
3. Resources and services that might be beneficial based on functional needs rather than diagnosis
4. Self-help strategies aligned with the identified pattern of strengths and challenges

This pragmatic focus ensures that assessment leads to practical benefit even when diagnostic certainty remains elusive.

Providing opportunity for reassessment acknowledges that diagnostic understanding may evolve with additional information or developmental changes. This might involve:

1. Discussing circumstances under which reassessment might be warranted
2. Identifying specific information that would help clarify diagnosis if it became available
3. Explaining how developmental changes or life transitions might reveal additional diagnostic information
4. Ensuring the individual knows how to access reassessment if needed in the future

This approach recognizes diagnostic assessment as an ongoing process rather than a one-time determination, particularly in complex or borderline cases.

Ethical considerations in managing diagnostic uncertainty include balancing several important principles:

Avoiding both over-diagnosis and under-diagnosis, as both can have negative consequences. Over-diagnosis may lead to inappropriate labelling, identity concerns, or unnecessary services, while under-diagnosis may prevent access to needed support, understanding, and accommodations. Navigating this balance requires careful weighing of the evidence, consideration of the potential benefits and harms of diagnosis for the specific individual, and transparent discussion of uncertainty.

Respecting the individual's perspective on their own experiences while maintaining diagnostic rigor. Many adults, seeking assessment, have conducted extensive research and strongly identify with autism descriptions. While this self-identification provides important information, it must be considered alongside objective assessment findings rather than determining diagnostic conclusions.

Respectful navigation of differences between self-perception and clinical assessment requires validation of the individual's experiences while maintaining professional integrity in diagnostic decision-making.

Considering access to support implications of diagnostic decisions, as formal diagnosis often serves as a gateway to services, accommodations, and benefits. When diagnosis is uncertain but support needs are clear, clinicians face ethical challenges in balancing diagnostic integrity with ensuring access to needed resources. Approaches might include:

1. Providing detailed functional assessment that documents support needs independent of diagnosis
2. Exploring alternative pathways to support that don't require definitive autism diagnosis
3. Offering provisional diagnosis with clear documentation of uncertainty when appropriate
4. Advocating for needs-based rather than diagnosis-based support systems

These approaches recognize the practical implications of diagnostic decisions while maintaining clinical integrity.

By developing sophisticated approaches to managing diagnostic uncertainty, clinicians can navigate complex presentations with appropriate caution while still providing meaningful understanding and support recommendations. This nuanced approach serves both the scientific integrity of diagnostic practice and the practical needs of individuals seeking assessment.

CHAPTER 33
Post-Diagnostic Support

Post-diagnostic support represents a critical component of comprehensive autism assessment services, bridging the gap between receiving a diagnosis and implementing effective strategies to enhance quality of life. Far from being an optional add-on, appropriate post-diagnostic support is essential for translating diagnostic understanding into meaningful life improvements. Without such support, diagnosis alone may provide explanation but fail to deliver practical benefit. Understanding the range of post-diagnostic needs and available support approaches allows clinicians to guide individuals toward resources and strategies most relevant to their specific profile and circumstances.

NHS Right to Choose discussions should form part of post-diagnostic planning, ensuring individuals are aware of their options for accessing support. Under the NHS Right to Choose framework, individuals have certain rights regarding where they receive healthcare, including some autism support services. Key points to discuss include:

1. Available NHS autism support services in the local area, including specialist teams, mental health services with autism expertise, and community support options
2. Waiting times and referral pathways for different service options
3. Circumstances under which individuals might choose alternative providers
4. Funding arrangements and potential limitations or exclusions
5. Process for exercising choice when options exist

This information empowers individuals to make informed decisions about their post-diagnostic support pathway, potentially reducing delays in accessing appropriate services.

Psychoeducation forms a foundation for post-diagnostic support, helping individuals develop accurate understanding of autism and its implications for their specific situation. Effective psychoeducation addresses:

Understanding autism as a neurodevelopmental condition, including:

1. Neurobiological basis of autism and its developmental nature
2. Current scientific understanding of autism's causes and mechanisms
3. Spectrum concept and the diversity of autism presentations
4. Distinction between autism and mental health conditions
5. Lifespan perspective on how autism features may evolve over time

This foundational knowledge helps counter misconceptions and provides a scientific framework for understanding personal experiences.

Strengths and differences framework emphasizes neurodiversity perspectives that recognize both the challenges associated with autism and the potential strengths and beneficial cognitive differences. This approach explores:

1. Common cognitive strengths associated with autism, such as attention to detail, pattern recognition, logical analysis, and long-term memory
2. How special interests can provide expertise, motivation, and potential career directions
3. Potential benefits of hyperfocus, persistence, and alternative perspective-taking
4. Understanding differences in social approach and communication style as variations rather than deficits
5. Recognition of genuine challenges while avoiding deficit-focused narratives

This balanced perspective supports positive identity development while acknowledging real-world challenges that may require support.

Individualized application of autism understanding involves connecting general information about autism to the person's specific experiences and challenges. This personalized approach explores:

1. How their unique profile of autism features affects daily functioning
2. Personal strengths and how these can be leveraged in different contexts
3. Specific challenges that have the greatest impact on quality of life
4. Historical experiences reinterpreted through the lens of autism understanding
5. Personal priorities for support and development

This individualized approach ensures that psychoeducation translates into personally relevant understanding rather than abstract knowledge.

Specific interventions may be recommended based on identified needs and preferences. While no interventions alter core autism features, many approaches can enhance skills, reduce distress, and improve quality of life:

Social skills development approaches may benefit individuals who wish to enhance their social communication abilities. These might include:

1. Social cognition training focusing on understanding social cues and perspectives
2. Conversation skills groups providing structured practice with feedback
3. Social problem-solving approaches addressing specific social challenges
4. Workplace social communication strategies for professional contexts
5. Dating and relationship skills programs for those interested in intimate relationships

These approaches should be offered as optional skill development rather than normalization efforts, respecting the individual's goals and preferences regarding social interaction.

Sensory management strategies address the significant impact sensory differences can have on daily functioning and wellbeing. Approaches might include:

1. Environmental modifications to reduce sensory overload at home, work, or educational settings
2. Sensory diet planning to ensure appropriate sensory input throughout the day
3. Techniques for managing unavoidable sensory challenges in public spaces
4. Sensory regulation strategies during periods of overload
5. Advocacy approaches for requesting sensory accommodations

These sensory-focused interventions often provide immediate quality of life improvements with relatively simple modifications and strategies.

Mental health support adapted for autism addresses the high rates of anxiety, depression, and other mental health conditions in the autistic population. This might include:

1. Cognitive-behavioural therapy adapted for autism, with adjustments for concrete thinking, executive functioning differences, and social cognition
2. Mindfulness approaches modified to accommodate sensory and attention differences
3. Emotion regulation strategies that consider alexithymia and interoceptive differences

4. Group therapy with others who share autism and mental health challenges
5. Medication management by professionals knowledgeable about autism presentations

These adapted mental health approaches recognize both the high prevalence of mental health challenges in autism and the need for autism-informed modifications to standard interventions.

Employment support addresses the significant vocational challenges many adults with autism experience despite strong capabilities in specific areas. This support might include:

1. Vocational assessment identifying strengths, challenges, and suitable work environments
2. Job coaching providing on-site support for workplace integration
3. Workplace accommodation planning and implementation
4. Disclosure decision-making support regarding if, when, and how to disclose autism
5. Self-advocacy skills for requesting needed adjustments and support

These employment-focused interventions aim to reduce the high rates of unemployment and underemployment in the autistic population by creating better matches between individual profiles and work environments.

Support networks play a crucial role in post-diagnostic adaptation and ongoing wellbeing. Information about various support options should be provided:

Local and national autism organizations offer various resources and services that should be discussed during post-diagnostic support planning:

The National Autistic Society: A Key Post-Diagnostic Resource

National Autistic Society provides comprehensive information, helpline services, advocacy support, and various local branches with specific services and activities. Their employment programs, legal rights information, and extensive online resources make them a key organization to highlight during post-diagnostic discussions.

Local autism services vary significantly across different UK regions but might include:

1. NHS specialist autism teams providing post-diagnostic support
2. Council-funded support services for adults with autism

3. Charitable organizations offering autism-specific programs
4. Peer support groups organized by local organizations
5. Social and activity groups designed for autistic adults

Providing specific information about local services, including referral processes, eligibility criteria, and waiting times, helps individuals navigate the often-complex service landscape.

Self-advocacy represents an essential skill for adults with autism, enabling them to effectively communicate their needs and secure appropriate accommodations across various life contexts. Support for developing self-advocacy skills might include:

- Understanding their rights under relevant legislation, particularly the **Equality Act 2010**, which establishes autism as a protected characteristic requiring reasonable adjustments in employment, education, and service provision
- Developing skills for explaining autism and specific support needs to others in clear, constructive ways
- Learning to identify and request specific accommodations that address individual challenges
- Practicing assertive communication for situations where needs are not being met
- Connecting with advocacy organizations that can provide additional support when needed

These self-advocacy skills enhance independence and ensure that diagnosis translates into practical accommodations across different environments.

UK resources for autistic adults should be highlighted during post-diagnostic support planning, providing accessible information about available support options:

NHS resources include:

1. Post-diagnostic information packs provided by many NHS autism assessment services
2. Local NHS autism support teams offering various post-diagnostic services
3. Autism-specific mental health pathways in some regions
4. Primary care annual health checks for adults with autism
5. Specialist NHS services for particular needs such as eating disorders or substance use with autism expertise

National organizations beyond the National Autistic Society include:

1. **Autistica**: Research charity providing evidence-based information and resources
2. **Autism Alliance**: Network of autism charities across the UK
3. **ARGH (Autistic Rights Group Highlands):** Autistic-led advocacy organization
4. **Resources for Autism**: Practical support services in some regions
5. **Ambitious About Autism**: Primarily youth-focused but with transition support for young adults

Local support groups provide opportunities for connection with others who share similar experiences. These might include:

1. Peer support groups facilitated by autistic adults
2. Special interest groups focusing on shared interests
3. Skills development groups addressing specific challenges
4. Social groups providing structured opportunities for connection
5. Online communities specific to local areas

Employment support resources include:

1. Access to Work: Government program funding workplace adjustments
2. Specialist employment agencies with autism expertise
3. Employers' autism networks in some regions
4. Supported internship programs for developing work skills
5. Career counselling services with autism knowledge

Educational support for those in further or higher education includes:

1. Disability services in universities and colleges
2. Disabled Students' Allowance funding support and accommodations
3. Study skills support adapted for autism-related learning differences
4. Examination arrangements accommodating sensory and executive functioning needs
5. Mentoring programs providing ongoing support throughout education

Benefits information should be provided regarding:

1. Personal Independence Payment eligibility and application process
2. Universal Credit considerations for autistic adults
3. Employment and Support Allowance for those unable to work

4. Council Tax reductions potentially available
5. Blue Badge eligibility for those with significant mobility challenges

Self-advocacy groups led by and for autistic individuals provide both practical support and connection with the broader autism community:

1. Autistic UK: National autistic-led organization
2. Local autistic-led groups across various UK regions
3. Online forums and social media communities
4. Advocacy collectives providing peer support for navigating services
5. Autistic speakers and consultants sharing lived experience perspectives

The implementation of post-diagnostic support faces several challenges in current UK service provision that should be acknowledged:

Service availability varies dramatically across different geographic regions, creating inequitable access to support. Some areas have comprehensive, well-resourced post-diagnostic services, while others offer minimal or no structured support following diagnosis. This "postcode lottery" means that individuals may need different levels of guidance and self-advocacy depending on their location.

Waiting times for post-diagnostic support can be substantial, sometimes extending to months or years for specific services. This delay between diagnosis and support can create significant difficulties during a critical period of adaptation and understanding. Clinicians should provide interim strategies and self-help resources to bridge these gaps when service delays are anticipated.

Funding constraints affect the availability, scope, and continuity of many post-diagnostic services. Time-limited funding models often lead to helpful programs being discontinued, while resource limitations may restrict eligibility criteria or session numbers below optimal levels. Understanding these constraints helps manage expectations and prioritize available resources effectively.

Despite these challenges, effective post-diagnostic support represents an essential component of the autism assessment pathway, translating diagnostic understanding into practical strategies that enhance quality of life and daily functioning. By providing comprehensive information about available resources and support approaches, clinicians help ensure that diagnosis serves as a gateway to appropriate support rather than simply providing a label without direction for moving forward.

CHAPTER 34

Pharmacological Considerations

While no medications directly treat core autism features, pharmacological interventions may play an important role in managing co-occurring conditions that frequently affect adults with autism. Understanding the evidence base, special considerations, and appropriate monitoring for medication use in the autistic population is essential for psychiatrists and other prescribers involved in autism care. This knowledge allows for thoughtful risk-benefit analysis and appropriate adaptation of standard approaches to address the unique needs and response patterns of autistic adults.

It is fundamental to emphasize that no medications currently treat core ASD symptoms. The primary autism features of social communication differences and restricted, repetitive patterns of behaviour do not respond to pharmacological intervention. This fact should be clearly communicated to individuals and families to prevent unrealistic expectations or inappropriate medication trials targeting these fundamental autism characteristics. The focus of pharmacological intervention should instead be on co-occurring conditions that may cause additional distress or functional impairment beyond core autism features.

Evidence-based approaches for comorbidities focus on several common co-occurring conditions that may benefit from medication management when appropriate:

Anxiety and depression occur at exceptionally high rates in the autistic population and may sometimes respond to pharmacological intervention. Medication approaches may include:

1. Selective serotonin reuptake inhibitors (SSRIs), which have shown effectiveness for anxiety and depression in some autistic adults, though response rates may differ from the general population
2. Serotonin-norepinephrine reuptake inhibitors (SNRIs) as an alternative for those who don't respond to or tolerate SSRIs
3. Buspirone for anxiety, particularly when SSRIs are contraindicated or poorly tolerated

4. Pregabalin or gabapentin for anxiety in some cases, particularly when physical symptoms predominate
5. Mirtazapine, which may be beneficial for those with both anxiety and sleep disturbance

When prescribing these medications, lower starting doses with more gradual titration is often necessary due to increased sensitivity to side effects. Additionally, careful monitoring for behavioural activation, increased agitation, or worsening of repetitive behaviours is important, as these adverse effects may be more common in the autistic population.

ADHD co-occurs in 30-50% of adults with autism and may significantly impact functioning. When ADHD symptoms cause impairment beyond what would be expected from autism alone, medication may be considered:

1. Methylphenidate has shown effectiveness for ADHD symptoms in autistic adults, with response rates similar to those in the general ADHD population, though side effect profiles may differ
2. Atomoxetine represents a non-stimulant option that may be effective, particularly when anxiety is a significant concern or when stimulants are contraindicated
3. Lisdexamfetamine and other amphetamine preparations may be options when methylphenidate is ineffective or poorly tolerated
4. Guanfacine extended-release has more limited evidence in adult populations but may be considered when other options are unsuccessful

Monitoring for both effectiveness and side effects should be particularly rigorous, as some autistic individuals may have difficulty identifying and communicating subjective medication effects. Standardized rating scales completed by both the individual and informants can provide more objective assessment of response.

Sleep disorders affect up to 80% of adults with autism and may significantly impact daytime functioning, mood, and behaviour. When behavioural and environmental approaches are insufficient, medication may be considered:

1. Melatonin has the strongest evidence base for autism-related sleep problems, with demonstrated effectiveness for sleep onset insomnia in particular. Extended-release formulations may help with sleep maintenance as well as initiation.
2. Sedating antihistamines are sometimes used but should be employed cautiously due to potential for tolerance, anticholinergic side effects, and limited evidence for long-term efficacy

3. Mirtazapine in low doses may be beneficial when sleep problems co-occur with anxiety or depression
4. Clonidine occasionally helps with sleep initiation, particularly when hyperarousal contributes to sleep difficulties
5. Z-drugs and benzodiazepines should generally be avoided due to risk of dependence and potential for paradoxical reactions

Sleep medication should always be prescribed alongside behavioural and environmental interventions rather than as standalone treatment.

Irritability and challenging behaviours may occasionally warrant pharmacological intervention when severe, persistent, and unresponsive to behavioural and environmental approaches. Medication considerations include:

1. Risperidone has the strongest evidence base for reducing severe irritability and challenging behaviours, though its significant side effect profile necessitates careful risk-benefit analysis
2. Aripiprazole also has demonstrated efficacy with potentially fewer metabolic side effects than risperidone, though other adverse effects like akathisia may be problematic
3. Mood stabilizers such as valproate may be considered in some cases, particularly when mood dysregulation appears to drive behavioural challenges
4. SSRIs might help when anxiety or obsessive-compulsive symptoms contribute to behavioural difficulties

These medications should be used judiciously, at the lowest effective dose, with regular reassessment of continuing need, and always as part of a comprehensive management approach that includes behavioural, environmental, and psychological interventions.

Considerations in ASD include several factors that may affect medication selection, dosing, and monitoring:

Potential for atypical responses to medication is well-documented in the autistic population. These atypical responses include:

1. Increased sensitivity to side effects, often requiring lower initial doses and more gradual titration than standard protocols
2. Paradoxical reactions, such as increased agitation with medications typically expected to reduce anxiety
3. Idiosyncratic responses not commonly seen in the general population

4. Different therapeutic dose ranges, sometimes requiring either unusually low or unusually high doses for effectiveness
5. Unexpected drug interactions that may not be well-documented in prescribing literature

These atypical responses necessitate individualized approaches to medication management rather than strict adherence to standard protocols.

Increased sensitivity to side effects represents a particularly important consideration in autism psychopharmacology. This heightened sensitivity may reflect several factors:

1. Altered drug metabolism due to genetic factors or co-occurring conditions
2. Different baseline neurochemistry affecting response to psychoactive compounds
3. Sensory hypersensitivities that amplify awareness of subtle bodily changes
4. Communication difficulties that may lead to distress from side effects that cannot be easily articulated

This increased sensitivity typically warrants a "start low, go slow" approach to medication initiation and titration, with smaller starting doses and more gradual increases than might be used in the general population.

Communication of adverse effects may be complicated by differences in interoception (awareness of internal bodily states), alexithymia (difficulty identifying and describing emotions), or expressive language limitations. These factors create challenges for standard medication monitoring that relies on spontaneous reporting of subjective side effects. Alternative monitoring approaches include:

1. Structured side effect checklists rather than open-ended questions
2. Visual analogy scales for rating symptom severity
3. Concrete, specific questioning about common side effects
4. Involvement of caregivers or support persons who may notice behavioural indicators of side effects
5. More frequent monitoring during medication initiation and dose changes

These adapted approaches help ensure that adverse effects are identified promptly despite potential communication barriers.

Monitoring challenges extend beyond side effect detection to assessment of therapeutic benefit. Standard approaches to evaluating medication effectiveness often rely on subjective reporting that may be difficult for some autistic individuals. Alternative monitoring strategies include:

1. Objective behavioural measures focusing on observable outcomes rather than subjective experiences
2. Frequency counts of specific target behaviours or symptoms
3. Functional assessments examining impact on daily activities and participation
4. Structured rating scales completed by both the individual and informants
5. Regular review of concrete goals established before medication initiation

These monitoring approaches provide more reliable assessment of medication effects than relying solely on general impressions or spontaneous reporting.

NICE guidance regarding medication use in autism emphasizes several key principles:

1. Medications should not be used to address core features of autism
2. Co-occurring conditions should be treated according to relevant clinical guidelines, with appropriate adaptations for autism
3. Specialist involvement is recommended when prescribing antipsychotics or other medications with significant risk profiles
4. Regular medication review should assess continuing need and monitor for adverse effects
5. Withdrawal of ineffective medications should be planned carefully with gradual tapering

These evidence-based recommendations provide a framework for appropriate medication use those balances potential benefits against risks.

The consent process for medication requires particular attention in autism care to ensure truly informed decision-making:

Accessible information about proposed medications should be provided in formats appropriate to the individual's information processing style. This might include:

1. Written information at appropriate reading level
2. Visual representations of key information
3. Concrete examples of potential benefits and side effects
4. Step-by-step explanation of monitoring procedures
5. Clear description of alternative options, including non-pharmacological approaches

This accessible information ensures that consent is based on genuine understanding rather than simply compliance with professional recommendations.

Decision-making capacity should be assessed thoughtfully, recognizing that autism itself does not imply incapacity but that some individuals may need support with specific aspects of medication decisions. Assessment should consider:

1. Ability to understand information about the proposed medication
2. Capacity to retain this information long enough to make a decision
3. Ability to weigh benefits against risks and side effects
4. Capability to communicate the decision by any means

When capacity is limited in some areas, appropriate decision-making supports should be provided rather than assuming complete incapacity.

Shared decision-making approaches are particularly valuable in autism pharmacology, involving collaborative discussion of:

1. The individual's goals and priorities for treatment
2. Potential benefits and risks of medication options
3. How success will be defined and measured
4. Timeframes for evaluating effectiveness
5. Circumstances under which medication would be discontinued

This collaborative approach respects autonomy while providing necessary clinical guidance for complex decisions.

Practical prescribing considerations for autistic adults include:

Medication selection factors extend beyond standard clinical guidelines to consider autism-specific issues such as:

1. Sensory sensitivities that might affect tolerance of medication formulations (taste, texture, smell)
2. Executive functioning challenges that could impact complex medication regimens
3. Co-occurring medical conditions that may influence medication choice
4. Previous medication experiences and preferences
5. Individual sensitivities to specific side effects based on sensory or anxiety profiles

These personalized considerations help identify medications most likely to be both effective and tolerable for the specific individual.

Formulation preferences may significantly affect medication adherence and tolerability. Important considerations include:

1. Difficulty swallowing tablets or capsules, which is common due to oral sensory sensitivities or coordination challenges
2. Taste and texture sensitivities that may make liquid formulations problematic
3. Preferences for specific colours, shapes, or sizes of tablets based on sensory profile
4. Need for consistent appearance of medications, as changes in generic formulations may cause distress
5. Ability to manage different formulation types within the context of daily routines

Discussing these preferences before prescribing can prevent adherence problems related to formulation aversions.

Timing and routine integration should be carefully planned, considering:

1. Existing daily routines and how medication can be incorporated without disruption
2. Optimal timing based on both pharmacokinetics and the individual's schedule
3. Strategies for remembering medication, which might include visual reminders, technology-based alerts, or incorporation into established routines
4. Plans for managing medication during routine changes, such as holidays or travel
5. Clear instructions for what to do if a dose is missed

This attention to practical implementation helps ensure that theoretically appropriate medication actually translates into real-world benefit.

The integration of pharmacological and non-pharmacological approaches represents best practice in autism care. Medication should be viewed as one component of a comprehensive support plan rather than a standalone intervention. This integrated approach includes:

1. Environmental modifications addressing sensory needs and predictability

2. Psychological therapies adapted for autism, such as modified cognitive-behavioural approaches
3. Skills development in areas of challenge, such as social communication or executive functioning
4. Support for daily living, education, or employment as needed
5. Regular review of how different interventions work together

This holistic approach recognizes that medication may address some symptoms while other supports target different aspects of functioning, creating a comprehensive support system tailored to individual needs.

CHAPTER 35

Assessment in Diverse Populations

Culturally competent autism assessment requires sophisticated understanding of how cultural factors influence the presentation, interpretation, and impact of autism features. The UK's diverse population necessitates assessment approaches that can distinguish between cultural differences and autism features while ensuring equitable access to diagnosis and support across different cultural contexts. Developing cultural competence in autism assessment involves recognizing the influence of culture on all aspects of the diagnostic process, from initial recognition of concerns to interpretation of assessment findings and development of support recommendations.

Cultural considerations significantly impact various aspects of autism assessment for example the cultural norms for social communication vary substantially across different cultural contexts, creating challenges for assessment of this core autism domain. These cultural variations include:

Eye contact norms that differ markedly across cultures. In many Western contexts, direct eye contact is expected during conversation and reduced eye contact may be interpreted as indicating social disinterest or difficulty. In contrast, in many East Asian, African, Middle Eastern, and Indigenous cultures, direct eye contact, particularly with authority figures or elders, may be considered disrespectful or inappropriate. These cultural differences in eye contact norms can lead to misinterpretation of culturally appropriate behaviour as autism-related social communication differences.

Conversational patterns also vary culturally, including turn-taking conventions, acceptable interruption patterns, use of silence, topic selection, and directness of communication. For example, some cultures value animated interruption as showing engagement, while others emphasize waiting for clear turn-taking signals. Similarly, Western communication often values direct statement of needs and opinions, while many Eastern cultures emphasize indirect communication that preserves harmony. These cultural differences in conversational style may be misinterpreted as pragmatic language difficulties associated with autism if not considered within their cultural context.

Nonverbal communication, including gesture use, physical proximity, and touch during interaction, is highly culturally determined. For instance, Mediterranean and Latin American cultures often involve more animated gesture and closer physical proximity than is typical in Northern European contexts. Facial expressiveness also varies culturally, with some cultures encouraging more animated display of emotion while others value emotional restraint. Without cultural context, these differences might be misinterpreted as unusual nonverbal communication associated with autism.

Social hierarchies and relationship expectations vary across cultures, influencing social behaviour in ways that may affect assessment. For example, some cultures emphasize deference to authority figures, including healthcare professionals, potentially affecting social presentation during assessment. Similarly, cultures differ in expectations regarding children's social roles, peer relationships, and participation in adult conversation, affecting developmental histories and current social expectations.

Assessment must carefully distinguish between culturally normative social communication patterns and those that reflect autism-related differences. This distinction requires knowledge of the specific cultural context, ideally through consultation with cultural informants when clinicians lack direct experience with the individual's cultural background.

Expression of emotions and distress also varies substantially across cultures, affecting both presentation and reporting of autism-related challenges:

Cultural display rules govern appropriate emotional expression, including which emotions may be openly expressed, in what contexts, and with what intensity. For example, some cultures emphasize emotional restraint and may discourage open expression of distress, while others encourage more expressive emotional communication. These cultural patterns influence how autism-related difficulties may be experienced and communicated.

Cultural idioms of distress refer to culture-specific ways of expressing psychological difficulty or suffering. For example, some cultures emphasize somatic complaints over emotional language when experiencing distress, while others may use culturally specific metaphors or explanatory frameworks. These cultural patterns may affect how autism-related challenges are described and conceptualized by individuals and families.

Help-seeking behaviour varies culturally, affecting when and how individuals access assessment services. Some cultural contexts emphasize self-reliance or family-based support rather than professional services, potentially delaying autism assessment. Other cultures may have specific pathways for addressing developmental or behavioural concerns that differ from mainstream healthcare systems. These cultural patterns influence the timing and context of assessment referrals.

Stigma related to developmental or mental health conditions varies across cultural contexts, potentially affecting willingness to seek assessment, disclose concerns, or accept diagnostic labels. In some cultural contexts, conditions affecting social functioning or behaviour may carry particularly significant stigma, creating barriers to autism assessment and support. Understanding and sensitively addressing these stigma concerns represents an important aspect of culturally competent assessment.

These cultural variations in emotional expression and distress communication require assessment approaches that are attuned to cultural context and avoid pathologizing culturally normative patterns while still identifying clinically significant autism features.

Family structures and expectations also vary culturally, influencing both the interpretation of development and the impact of potential autism features:

Developmental expectations vary across cultures, including expectations for developmental milestones, appropriate child behaviour, and independence development. For example, some cultures expect earlier development of self-care skills while others emphasize academic achievement or social behaviour. These varying expectations influence when developmental differences raise concern and how they are interpreted.

Child-rearing practices differ substantially across cultures, including approaches to discipline, communication with children, play expectations, and independence fostering. These cultural patterns affect both the developmental environment and the interpretation of child behaviour, potentially influencing the expression and recognition of autism features.

Family involvement in assessment may follow different cultural patterns, affecting who participates, how information is shared, and who makes decisions about assessment and support. In some cultures, extended family members play significant roles in child-related decisions, while others emphasize nuclear family or individual autonomy. Culturally competent assessment accommodates these different family structures and decision-making patterns.

Cultural concepts of development and disability influence how autism-related behaviours are understood and explained. Some cultural traditions have specific frameworks for understanding developmental differences that may align with or differ from Western medical models. These cultural conceptualizations influence how assessment information is received and integrated into the family's understanding.

Sensitivity to these cultural variations in family structure and expectations supports more accurate assessment and more effective engagement with individuals and families from diverse cultural backgrounds.

Socioeconomic factors often intersect with cultural considerations, creating complex influences on the assessment process:

Access to healthcare and education varies significantly across different socioeconomic groups, affecting previous identification of developmental concerns, availability of developmental records, and familiarity with assessment processes. Limited access to healthcare may result in delayed recognition of developmental differences, while educational disadvantage may affect performance on standardized measures.

Historical documentation availability may be limited for individuals from refugee backgrounds, those who have experienced frequent relocations, or those educated in settings with limited record-keeping. This documentation gap creates challenges for developmental history assessment and may require greater reliance on current observation and creative approaches to historical information gathering.

Socioeconomic stressors may influence both the expression and impact of autism features, as financial hardship, housing instability, or food insecurity create additional challenges that may exacerbate or mask autism-related difficulties. Assessment must consider these contextual factors in interpreting presenting concerns and functional impact.

Migration experiences create additional layers of complexity, as individuals may have developed in one cultural context but currently live in another. This bicultural experience may involve navigating different social expectations across contexts, potential language barriers, and adaptation to new systems and structures. Assessment must consider both original and current cultural contexts in interpreting development and current functioning.

These socioeconomic factors require assessment approaches that consider the broader social determinants of health and development rather than viewing autism features in isolation from their socioeconomic context.

Language differences present particular challenges for autism assessment, as many standardized measures and interview approaches assume fluency in the assessment language:

Assessment in non-native language significantly disadvantages individuals being assessed in a language other than their first language. Even those with good conversational skills in the assessment language may struggle with the cognitive and linguistic demands of standardized measures, potentially underperforming relative to their true abilities. Similarly, subtle pragmatic language differences may be difficult to distinguish from second language acquisition patterns.

Use of interpreters introduces additional complexity to the assessment process. While essential for accurate communication, interpreter-mediated assessment involves potential challenges including:

1. Loss of subtle linguistic and pragmatic features through translation
2. Cultural differences in understanding of assessment questions and concepts
3. Potential discomfort discussing sensitive topics through a third party
4. Logistical complexities of coordinating assessment with interpreter availability

Effective interpreter-mediated assessment requires specific adaptations, including:

1. Briefing interpreters about the assessment purpose and approach
2. Allowing additional time for translated communication
3. Using simple, concrete language that translates more accurately
4. Checking understanding frequently through various means
5. Considering cultural factors that may influence interpreter-individual interaction

Validity of standardized measures becomes particularly problematic when assessing individuals from cultural and linguistic backgrounds different from the normative samples. Most autism assessment measures were developed and validated primarily with white, Western, English-speaking populations, creating potential bias when applied in different cultural contexts. This limitation requires cautious interpretation of standardized results and greater reliance on clinical judgment informed by cultural consultation.

UK context presents specific diversity considerations reflecting the nation's multicultural population:

Diverse population needs within the NHS require service adaptations to ensure equitable access and appropriate assessment. The UK's population includes significant communities from **South Asian, African, Caribbean, Eastern European, Middle Eastern, and East Asian backgrounds**, among others, each with distinct cultural perspectives relevant to autism assessment. Additionally, the UK includes indigenous cultural differences, with Welsh, Scottish, and Northern Irish cultural contexts that may differ from English norms.

Regional variations in cultural diversity mean that services in different areas may need different cultural competence priorities based on local population demographics. Urban centres typically have greater cultural diversity requiring broader cultural knowledge, while some regions have specific large cultural communities requiring in-depth understanding of particular cultural contexts.

Religious diversity intersects with cultural factors, as religious beliefs and practices may influence understanding of development, help-seeking behaviour, and family decision-making. Major faith communities in the UK include various Christian denominations, Islam, Hinduism, Sikhism, Judaism, and Buddhism, each with potential influences on how autism features are understood and addressed.

Migration patterns continue to evolve, requiring ongoing development of cultural competence for newly arriving communities. Recent years have seen significant migration from Eastern Europe, the Middle East, and parts of Africa, necessitating development of assessment approaches appropriate for these cultural contexts.

These UK-specific diversity considerations require both broad cultural competence principles and specific knowledge relevant to major cultural communities within the UK context.

Adaptations to standard assessment approaches are essential for culturally sensitive and valid assessment:

Cultural consultants can provide valuable expertise when assessing individuals from cultural backgrounds unfamiliar to the clinician. These consultants might include:

1. Clinicians from the relevant cultural background
2. Cultural liaison professionals within healthcare services
3. Community leaders or educators from the cultural group
4. Academic experts in cross-cultural aspects of autism
5. Autistic individuals from the relevant cultural background

These consultants can provide guidance on interpreting behaviours within cultural context, adapting assessment approaches appropriately, and developing culturally relevant support recommendations.

Adapted assessment materials may be necessary when standard measures are culturally inappropriate or unavailable in the required language. Adaptations might include:

1. Culturally modified versions of standardized instruments, when available
2. Translation of key measures with cultural adaptation rather than literal translation
3. Development of culturally specific behavioural observations focusing on features that transcend cultural boundaries
4. Use of local norms when available rather than Western standardization samples
5. Greater emphasis on functional assessment relative to standardized testing

These adapted approaches prioritize valid assessment over strict adherence to standardized protocols that may be culturally biased.

Flexible approaches to gathering developmental history may be necessary when standard history-taking methods are culturally inappropriate or when historical documentation is limited. Alternative approaches might include:

1. Group family interviews when collective information-sharing is culturally preferred
2. Use of photographic or video records to prompt recall and discussion
3. Timeline approaches that reference major cultural or community events
4. Exploration of development through cultural frameworks meaningful to the family
5. Greater emphasis on current functioning when historical information remains limited despite alternative approaches

These flexible history-gathering methods recognize that standard Western clinical interviewing may not be optimal for all cultural contexts.

Community engagement approaches may enhance assessment and support planning by involving cultural community resources. These approaches might include:

1. Collaboration with cultural community organizations in developing assessment and support services
2. Incorporation of community perspectives on disability and support
3. Partnership with cultural community leaders in service planning and delivery

4. Development of culturally specific post-diagnostic support options
5. Training and employment of staff from diverse cultural backgrounds

These community engagement strategies recognize that culturally appropriate services require ongoing partnership rather than simply modified assessment techniques.

Developing cultural competence requires specific approaches to professional development and service design:

Training for clinicians should address both general cultural competence principles and specific knowledge about major cultural groups within the service area. Effective training approaches include:

1. Didactic education about cultural variations relevant to autism assessment
2. Case-based learning exploring cultural complexity in assessment
3. Reflective practice examining personal cultural assumptions and biases
4. Direct learning from autistic individuals from diverse cultural backgrounds
5. Ongoing supervision addressing cultural aspects of assessment

This comprehensive training approach recognizes that cultural competence represents an ongoing developmental process rather than a fixed skill set.

Service design should incorporate cultural considerations from the outset rather than as an afterthought. Culturally competent service design includes:

1. Diverse staffing reflecting the cultural composition of the service population
2. Readily available interpreter services with interpreters trained in autism assessment
3. Flexible appointment structures accommodating different cultural approaches to healthcare
4. Assessment materials available in major community languages
5. Engagement with cultural community organizations in service planning and evaluation.

CHAPTER 36

Ethical Considerations

Autism assessment involves numerous ethical dimensions that require careful consideration to ensure practice that respects individual rights, promotes wellbeing, and adheres to professional ethical standards. Clinicians must navigate complex ethical terrain, balancing competing considerations such as diagnostic accuracy, individual preferences, access to support, and potential stigma. Understanding these ethical dimensions is essential for assessment that is not only technically sound but ethically robust.

Diagnostic disclosure represents a fundamental ethical consideration in autism assessment, requiring thoughtful approaches that balance multiple factors:

Benefits of diagnosis include providing an explanatory framework for lifelong experiences, potentially enhancing self-understanding and reducing self-blame for difficulties. Diagnosis may also facilitate access to support services, workplace or educational accommodations, and connections with the autism community. For many adults, diagnosis validates experiences and challenges that may previously have been misunderstood or dismissed.

Challenges following diagnosis may include adjustment to a new understanding of self, potential stigma or discrimination, and practical concerns about disclosure to others. Some individuals may experience grief related to late identification or worry about future implications of the diagnosis. The diagnosis may also lead to complex identity questions as the person integrates this new understanding into their self-concept.

The ethics of disclosure involve balancing these potential benefits and challenges while respecting individual autonomy in the diagnostic process. Key ethical principles include:

1. Respect for the individual's right to information about themselves and their neurodevelopment
2. Non-maleficence, considering potential harms associated with both diagnosis and non-diagnosis

3. Beneficence, focusing on how diagnosis can support wellbeing and development
4. Justice, ensuring equitable access to accurate diagnosis regardless of background or circumstances

These ethical principles guide approaches to diagnostic disclosure that maximize benefit while minimizing potential harm.

The disclosure process should be tailored to the individual's needs, preferences, and circumstances. Ethical disclosure involves:

1. Clear, honest communication of diagnostic conclusions using language appropriate to the individual's understanding.
2. Explanation of the basis for diagnostic decisions, including the specific evidence supporting the diagnosis.
3. Balanced discussion of what the diagnosis means, avoiding both overly negative framing and unrealistic positivity.
4. Recognition of the emotional impact of diagnosis and provision of appropriate support for processing this information.
5. Respect for the individual's pace in absorbing and responding to diagnostic information.

This individualized approach to disclosure recognizes that while all individuals have the right to information about their own diagnosis, how that information is shared should be adapted to their specific needs and context.

Capacity and consent considerations are particularly important in adult autism assessment, as they directly impact individual autonomy and rights:

Ensuring informed consent for assessment requires that individuals understand the nature and purpose of the assessment process, the information that will be gathered, potential outcomes, and how assessment information will be used. This informed consent is fundamental to ethical practice and requires:

1. Clear explanation of the assessment process in language the individual can understand.
2. Discussion of potential benefits and risks of assessment.
3. Explanation of confidentiality and its limits.
4. Information about how assessment findings will be documented and shared.
5. Recognition that consent is an ongoing process that can be withdrawn at any point.

These consent processes should be adapted to accommodate communication differences associated with autism, potentially including written information, visual supports, or involvement of advocates when helpful.

Assessment of decision-making capacity represents an important ethical consideration when individuals have cognitive or communication differences that might affect understanding or decision-making. Capacity assessment should:

1. Focus on specific decisions rather than global capacity.
2. Assess understanding of relevant information, ability to retain and weigh this information, and ability to communicate decisions.
3. Provide appropriate support to maximize capacity before concluding that capacity is lacking.
4. Consider the complexity of the specific decision rather than applying a one-size-fits-all approach.

When capacity is determined to be lacking for specific assessment-related decisions, appropriate safeguards should be implemented to protect the individual's rights and interests.

Adaptations to support informed consent and decision-making may include:

1. Simplified language explaining assessment procedures and implications.
2. Visual supports illustrating the assessment process and potential outcomes.
3. Extended time for processing information and making decisions.
4. Breaking complex decisions into smaller, more manageable components.
5. Involvement of advocates or supporters who understand the individual's communication style and preferences.

These adaptations help ensure that communication or cognitive differences do not unnecessarily limit autonomy in the assessment process.

Confidentiality and information sharing present complex ethical considerations in autism assessment, particularly regarding the involvement of family members, partners, or carers.

Balancing privacy with support needs requires careful navigation of sometimes competing considerations. While respecting confidentiality is a fundamental ethical principle, many adults with autism benefit from involvement of support persons in aspects of the assessment process. Ethical approaches to this balance include:

1. Explicit discussion of confidentiality parameters at the outset of assessment.
2. Clear consent processes for sharing information with specific individuals.
3. Consideration of capacity when determining appropriate information sharing.
4. Differentiated consent for different types of information or different support persons.
5. Regular review of information sharing preferences as the assessment progresses.

These approaches prioritize individual autonomy in information sharing decisions while recognizing the potential value of appropriate supporter involvement.

Legal frameworks governing information sharing in the UK include:

1. The **General Data Protection Regulation (GDPR)** and **Data Protection Act 2018**, which establish principles for processing personal data, including health information.
2. The **Mental Capacity Act 2005**, which provides frameworks for decision-making when capacity is lacking.
3. Professional codes of ethics from relevant bodies such as the **General Medical Council, British Psychological Society, or Royal College of Psychiatrists.**
4. NHS information governance policies that establish standards for handling patient information.

These legal and policy frameworks provide boundaries within which clinical judgment must operate regarding information sharing decisions.

Practical approaches to managing information sharing ethically include:

1. Separating assessment components that require family/informant input from those that can remain private.
2. Offering individuals the opportunity to review and comment on informant-provided information.
3. Providing different levels of detail in different documentation based on its intended audience and purpose.
4. Developing protocols for managing disagreements between self-report and informant report.
5. Creating opportunities for collaborative information sharing through joint feedback sessions when appropriate.

These practical approaches allow for beneficial information sharing while preserving privacy and autonomy to the greatest extent possible.

Access to services and equity considerations represent important ethical dimensions of autism assessment.

Often these barriers to diagnosis disproportionately affect certain populations, creating inequitable access to appropriate assessment and support. These barriers include:

1. Geographic disparities in service availability, with rural areas often having limited specialized assessment services.
2. Socioeconomic barriers including transportation costs, inability to take time off work, or lack of childcare during assessment.
3. Cultural and linguistic barriers affecting both referral patterns and assessment validity.
4. Gender biases leading to underdiagnosis in females and gender-diverse individuals.
5. Age-related barriers, with older adults often facing greater challenges accessing appropriate assessment.

Addressing these barriers represents an ethical imperative grounded in principles of justice and equal access to healthcare.

Waitlist management ethics become relevant when demand for assessment services exceeds capacity, creating sometimes lengthy waiting periods. Ethical approaches to waitlist management include:

1. Clear, transparent criteria for prioritization that balance clinical need, risk, and waiting time.
2. Interim support options for those waiting for full assessment.
3. Regular review of waiting individuals to identify changing circumstances that might affect prioritization.
4. System-level advocacy for increased assessment capacity rather than simply managing limited resources.
5. Consideration of alternative service models that might reduce waiting times.

These approaches aim to balance competing ethical considerations when resource constraints prevent immediate assessment for all who need it.

Advocacy for equitable service provision represents an ethical responsibility for clinicians involved in autism assessment. This advocacy might include:

1. Documenting unmet needs and service gaps to inform commissioning and service planning.
2. Developing innovative service models to address access barriers.
3. Training colleagues in recognition of autism across diverse presentations.
4. Participating in service improvement initiatives addressing equity issues.
5. Supporting self-advocacy and service user involvement in service development.

This advocacy extends professional ethics beyond individual clinical interactions to systemic change that promotes more equitable access.

Stigma and discrimination concerns must be considered throughout the assessment process.

Impact of diagnostic labels varies across individuals and contexts. While diagnosis often provides helpful explanation and access to support, it may also expose individuals to stigma or discrimination in some contexts. Ethical practice involves:

1. Discussing potential implications of diagnosis for different life domains.
2. Providing guidance on disclosure decisions in various contexts.
3. Ensuring diagnostic documentation serves beneficial purposes without unnecessarily labelling.
4. Using respectful, non-stigmatizing language in all assessment documentation.
5. Explicitly addressing strengths and capabilities alongside challenges.

This balanced approach recognizes both the potential benefits and risks associated with diagnostic labels.

Supporting against disadvantage involves going beyond diagnosis to address potential discrimination or barriers. This support might include:

1. Education about rights under the **Equality Act 2010**, which establishes autism as a protected characteristic.
2. Information about challenging discrimination in employment, education, or service provision.
3. Connections with advocacy organizations that can provide ongoing support.
4. Practical strategies for requesting and implementing reasonable adjustments.
5. Development of self-advocacy skills for navigating potentially discriminatory situations.

This support helps translate diagnostic information into practical protection against disadvantage.

Educational and workplace considerations deserve particular attention, as these represent domains where both support benefits and potential discrimination risks are significant. Ethical practice includes:

1. Careful consideration of how diagnostic information is shared with educational institutions or employers.
2. Focus on specific support needs and adjustments rather than diagnostic labels alone.
3. Emphasis on capabilities and potential alongside support needs.
4. Balanced documentation that facilitates appropriate accommodations without unnecessarily highlighting differences.
5. Ongoing availability for consultation regarding reasonable adjustments.

This approach maximizes the benefit of diagnosis in these key life domains while minimizing potential stigma or discrimination.

Neurodiversity perspective versus medical model considerations reflects broader ethical questions about how autism is conceptualized and approached.

Respect for difference versus pathologization represents a central ethical tension in autism assessment. The neurodiversity paradigm views autism as a natural variation in human neurocognitive functioning rather than inherently a disorder or deficit. This perspective emphasizes:

1. Recognition of autism as a different, not lesser, way of experiencing and interacting with the world.
2. Appreciation of cognitive strengths and differences that may accompany autism.
3. Focus on environmental barriers and accommodations rather than "fixing" the individual.
4. Respect for autistic identity and culture.
5. Recognition that many autism-related challenges reflect poor environmental fit rather than inherent deficits.

Balancing this perspective with recognition of genuine support needs that may benefit from a more medical framework requires nuanced ethical judgment.

Language and framing significantly impact how autism is understood and experienced. Ethical considerations include:

1. Respect for individual preferences regarding identity-first language ("autistic person") versus person-first language ("person with autism".)
2. Avoidance of deficit-focused or pathologizing language in assessment documentation.
3. Balance between acknowledging challenges and recognizing strengths and differences.
4. Consideration of how diagnostic language may be interpreted by the individual and others.
5. Awareness of the power of professional language to shape self-concept and others' perceptions.

These language considerations influence how diagnostic information affects self-understanding and social responses.

UK legal framework relevant to ethical practice in autism assessment includes:

Equality Act 2010 that establishes autism as a protected characteristic, providing legal protection against discrimination in employment, education, and service provision. This legal framework:

1. Establishes the right to reasonable adjustments in workplaces, educational settings, and services
2. Prohibits direct and indirect discrimination related to autism
3. Provides legal recourse when discrimination occurs
4. Creates obligations for organizations to proactively consider accessibility needs
5. Establishes autism as a disability for legal purposes regardless of severity or presentation

Understanding this legal framework helps clinicians support individuals in accessing appropriate protections following diagnosis.

Mental Capacity Act 2005 which provides the legal framework for assessing capacity and making decisions in the best interests of those lacking capacity for specific decisions. This legislation:

1. Establishes the presumption of capacity and the obligation to support decision-making
2. Provides a framework for assessing capacity when concerns arise
3. Establishes principles for best-interests decision-making when capacity is lacking

4. Creates protective mechanisms including Independent Mental Capacity Advocates
5. Guides practice regarding consent and decision-making throughout the assessment process

This legal framework shapes ethical practice regarding consent, capacity, and decision-making in the assessment context.

Professional ethical codes from relevant bodies provide additional guidance for ethical practice in autism assessment:

1. General Medical Council guidance on consent, confidentiality, and professional conduct
2. British Psychological Society Code of Ethics and Conduct
3. Royal College of Psychiatrists ethical guidance
4. Health and Care Professions Council Standards of Conduct, Performance and Ethics
5. Nursing and Midwifery Council Code of Professional Standards

These professional frameworks establish expectations for ethical practice that complement legal requirements and apply specifically to different professional groups involved in autism assessment.

By navigating these various ethical dimensions thoughtfully, clinicians can ensure that autism assessment not only meets technical standards but upholds fundamental ethical principles of respect for autonomy, beneficence, non-maleficence, and justice.

CHAPTER 37

Remote Assessment Considerations

The COVID-19 pandemic accelerated the development and implementation of remote assessment approaches for autism, creating both opportunities and challenges for clinical practice. While initially developed as a necessity during pandemic restrictions, telehealth options for various components of autism assessment have demonstrated potential benefits that extend beyond the pandemic context. Understanding the evidence base, limitations, technological requirements, and best practices for remote assessment is essential for determining when this approach may be appropriate and how it can be implemented effectively while maintaining assessment quality and validity.

The pandemic impact on autism assessment services was profound, necessitating rapid adaptation of previously in-person assessment models. This impact included shift toward telehealth options as in-person services were restricted or suspended during lockdown periods. This rapid transition required:

1. Development of new assessment protocols adapted for remote delivery
2. Training for clinicians in telehealth platforms and remote assessment techniques
3. Adaptation of standardized assessment instruments for virtual administration
4. New approaches to gathering observational data without direct in-person contact
5. Modified consent processes addressing the specific considerations of remote assessment

This shift represented an unprecedented change in standard practice, driven by the necessity to maintain some level of service provision despite physical distancing requirements.

Service disruptions and increased waiting times resulted from both the suspension of services during acute pandemic phases and the reduced efficiency of newly implemented remote processes. These disruptions created:

1. Extended waitlists as assessment capacity decreased while referrals continued or increased
2. Incomplete assessments when certain components could not be adequately adapted for remote delivery
3. Delayed diagnoses and subsequent support implementation
4. Increased distress for individuals and families awaiting assessment
5. Pressure to develop innovative solutions to address growing unmet needs

These service challenges prompted critical examination of assessment models and exploration of alternative approaches that could maintain service provision during periods of restriction.

Innovation and adaptation emerged from this challenging context, as services developed creative solutions to assessment barriers. These innovations included:

1. Hybrid assessment models combining remote and in-person elements
2. Greater emphasis on pre-assessment information gathering to maximize efficiency of direct assessment
3. New approaches to observational assessment using video recordings or structured remote activities
4. Enhanced roles for local professionals working under the guidance of specialist teams
5. Increased involvement of families in structured observation and data collection

Many of these innovations have continued relevance in post-pandemic practice, offering potential benefits for service efficiency and accessibility beyond the original crisis context.

The evidence base for remote assessment has developed significantly since the early pandemic period, providing better understanding of its validity and limitations.

Growing research on validity has examined the comparability of remote and in-person assessment findings. Key research findings include:

1. Good agreement between remote and in-person cognitive assessments for individuals with adequate verbal abilities and attention
2. Acceptable reliability for certain components of standardized autism assessments when adapted for remote administration
3. High satisfaction rates among many service users regarding remote assessment experiences

4. Comparable diagnostic conclusions in many cases, particularly for clear-cut presentations
5. Specific challenges in remote assessment of nonverbal communication, subtle social cues, and sensory behaviour's

This research suggests that while remote assessment has limitations, it may provide valid information for certain individuals and assessment components when properly implemented.

Technology-mediated assessment presents both opportunities and challenges for specific autism features:

1. Social communication assessment via videoconferencing captures many aspects of verbal communication but may miss subtle nonverbal cues, particularly eye contact patterns and peripheral movements
2. Restricted and repetitive behaviour's may be partially observable but with limited ability to assess environmental interactions or sensory seeking behaviour's
3. Cognitive assessment can be conducted remotely with adequate validity for many abilities, though manipulative tasks and processing speed assessment present greater challenges
4. History-taking and interviewing generally translate well to remote formats, sometimes with improved attendance and engagement
5. Standardized measures vary in their adaptability to remote administration, with some requiring significant modification

Understanding these domain-specific considerations helps determine which assessment components may be appropriate for remote delivery for particular individuals.

The development of telehealth-specific protocols has enhanced the validity of remote assessment:

1. Modified administration procedures for standardized instruments, with publisher-approved adaptations for remote delivery
2. Structured observation protocols designed specifically for videoconferencing contexts
3. Guidelines for environmental setup to optimize observational quality
4. Methods for remote collaboration with local professionals to supplement videoconferencing assessment
5. Approaches for incorporating pre-recorded video of naturalistic behaviour into assessment

These specialized protocols acknowledge the unique characteristics of remote assessment rather than simply attempting to replicate in-person procedures in a virtual environment.

Appropriate candidates for remote assessment may include:

Verbal, technology-capable individuals typically represent the most appropriate candidates for significant remote assessment components. Suitable individuals generally have:

1. Functional verbal communication allowing engagement in interview and discussion
2. Sufficient attention span to maintain focus during videoconferencing sessions
3. Adequate hearing and vision to engage with remote technology
4. Access to appropriate technology and internet connectivity
5. Comfort with technology-mediated interaction

For individuals with these characteristics, remote assessment components may provide valid information while potentially improving accessibility and efficiency.

Caregiver availability and engagement becomes particularly important in remote assessment contexts. Beneficial caregiver involvement includes:

1. Assistance with technology setup and troubleshooting
2. Creation of appropriate assessment environment with minimal distractions
3. Facilitation of structured activities for remote observation
4. Provision of collateral information about functioning in daily contexts
5. Support for the individual's engagement throughout the assessment process

This caregiver involvement must be balanced with appropriate independence for adult assessment, but some level of support typically enhances the quality of remote assessment data.

Stable home environment with adequate privacy and minimal distractions supports effective remote assessment. Important environmental factors include:

1. Private space where confidential discussions can occur without interruption
2. Adequate lighting for clear visual observation
3. Stable internet connection with sufficient bandwidth for videoconferencing
4. Minimal background noise that might interfere with communication

5. Appropriate seating and positioning for extended screen-based interaction

When these environmental conditions cannot be established in the home, alternative locations such as local healthcare facilities, community centres, or educational settings might be considered for remote connection to specialist assessors.

Limitations of remote assessment must be carefully considered when determining its appropriateness.

Observation constraints represent perhaps the most significant limitation of remote assessment approaches. These constraints include:

1. Limited field of view capturing only what appears on camera, potentially missing whole-body movements, environmental interactions, or off-camera behaviour's
2. Reduced ability to observe subtle nonverbal cues such as small changes in facial expression or brief gestures
3. Two-dimensional viewing that may obscure depth cues relevant to personal space and physical positioning
4. Inability to observe interactions with the physical environment and sensory responses to environmental stimuli
5. Technical issues such as poor video quality, lag, or freezing that interrupt behavioural observation

These observational limitations may be particularly significant when assessing individuals with subtle presentations or complex diagnostic questions.

Nonverbal cue assessment presents specific challenges in remote contexts. Difficulties include:

1. Altered eye contact patterns in videoconferencing, where looking at the camera rather than the screen creates the appearance of eye contact
2. Limited ability to observe peripheral nonverbal communication while maintaining engagement
3. Technology effects on prosody and timing of speech, potentially affecting assessment of communication rhythm
4. Reduced observation of body language and posture beyond what is visible on camera
5. Difficulty assessing interpersonal spacing and physical boundaries in virtual interaction

These challenges in nonverbal assessment may reduce confidence in diagnostic decisions, particularly for individuals whose autism features manifest primarily through subtle nonverbal communication differences.

Standardized testing challenges in remote delivery include:

1. Inability to control the testing environment completely, potentially affecting standardization
2. Difficulties administering timed tests with precise timing
3. Limited ability to observe problem-solving approaches and strategies
4. Challenges presenting visual or manipulative materials with consistent positioning and visibility
5. Potential for technological interruptions affecting test performance

These standardization concerns may be particularly significant for cognitive assessment components, where precise administration procedures are essential for valid interpretation.

Technical issues affecting assessment quality might include:

1. Poor internet connectivity causing video freezing, audio delays, or disconnection
2. Inadequate equipment such as low-quality cameras or microphones
3. Platform limitations in screen sharing, recording, or interaction capabilities
4. Variable technology skills among both clinicians and service users
5. Security and privacy concerns with various telehealth platforms

These technical challenges can significantly impact assessment quality and must be addressed through both technical solutions and procedural adaptations.

UK guidance regarding remote assessment has evolved throughout the pandemic period.

NHS Digital guidance has addressed various aspects of remote assessment implementation, including:

1. Information governance requirements for telehealth platforms
2. Consent procedures specific to remote assessment
3. Risk assessment for remote versus in-person service delivery
4. Technical specifications for healthcare videoconferencing
5. Documentation standards for remotely delivered assessment

This guidance provides a framework for implementing remote assessment components within NHS settings, addressing both clinical and governance considerations.

Royal College position statements from various professional bodies have addressed remote assessment considerations. These statements typically:

1. Acknowledge the necessity of remote options in certain circumstances
2. Emphasize the importance of clinical judgment in determining appropriateness
3. Highlight limitations and the need for in-person components when essential
4. Address training needs for clinicians delivering remote assessment
5. Call for ongoing research regarding validity and best practices

These professional guidelines provide important context for clinical decision-making regarding remote assessment implementation.

Local trust policies have been developed to operationalize national guidance within specific service contexts. These policies typically address:

1. Specific approved platforms for clinical videoconferencing
2. Technical support resources for staff and service users
3. Procedures for managing risk or technical failures during remote sessions
4. Documentation requirements specific to remote assessment
5. Integration of remote and in-person components in hybrid assessment models

Familiarity with these local policies is essential for clinicians implementing remote assessment components within NHS settings.

Hybrid approaches combining remote and in-person elements have emerged as promising models that leverage the benefits of remote assessment while addressing its limitations.

Combined remote and in-person elements might include:

1. Remote history-taking and interviewing to maximize efficiency of in-person time
2. In-person observational assessment and standardized testing requiring physical presence
3. Remote follow-up to discuss findings and recommendations after in-person assessment

4. Collaboration between remote specialist teams and local professionals who can conduct in-person components
5. Remote pre-assessment screening to determine appropriateness of full assessment

These hybrid approaches recognize that different assessment components vary in their suitability for remote delivery, allowing for tailored combinations that optimize both validity and efficiency.

Technical requirements for effective remote assessment include:

Secure platforms compliant with healthcare information governance requirements that are essential for clinical videoconferencing. Important platform considerations include:

1. End-to-end encryption of video and audio data
2. Compliance with relevant data protection regulations including GDPR
3. Authentication procedures ensuring session security
4. Controlled access preventing unauthorized participation
5. Appropriate data storage and management practices

NHS organizations typically specify approved platforms that meet these security requirements, such as Attend Anywhere, MS Teams for Healthcare, or certain configurations of Zoom Healthcare.

Connectivity requirements for quality assessment include:

1. Sufficient bandwidth for stable, high-quality video (typically minimum 1.5 Mbps upload/download)
2. Reliable internet connection with minimal interruption
3. Wired connections when possible, or strong Wi-Fi signal
4. Backup options for connection failures, such as phone availability
5. Technical support resources for troubleshooting connection issues

These connectivity requirements may present barriers for individuals in areas with limited internet infrastructure or those experiencing digital poverty, creating potential equity concerns for remote assessment approaches.

Equipment specifications for optimal assessment include:

1. Cameras with sufficient resolution for clear observation (minimum 720p HD)
2. Quality microphones capturing clear audio without significant background noise

3. Screens large enough to observe facial expressions and demonstrations
4. Positioning flexibility to adjust camera angles for different assessment activities
5. Lighting adequate for clear visibility of facial expressions and movements

While professional-grade equipment enhances assessment quality, the rapidly improving quality of consumer technology means that many standard laptops, tablets, or smartphones may provide adequate capabilities for certain assessment components.

Privacy considerations specific to remote assessment include:

1. Private physical spaces for both clinician and individual during videoconferencing
2. Secure, professional platforms rather than consumer social media or messaging apps
3. Clear information about recording practices and data storage
4. Protocols for managing sensitive discussions when privacy cannot be guaranteed
5. Alternative approaches when adequate privacy cannot be established

These privacy considerations are particularly important when assessing adults who may be discussing sensitive personal information and require confidential assessment environments.

Remote assessment approaches thus offer both valuable opportunities for increasing assessment accessibility and efficiency and significant limitations that must be carefully considered in determining their appropriate implementation. By understanding both the potential and constraints of remote assessment, clinicians can make informed decisions about when and how to incorporate these approaches into comprehensive autism assessment services.

CHAPTER 38

Complex Case Examples - Case 1

Examining complex case examples provides valuable opportunities to apply assessment principles to challenging clinical presentations. These examples illustrate the nuanced clinical decision-making required when autism features interact with other factors such as gender, mental health conditions, compensatory strategies, or limited developmental information. By analysing these complex cases, clinicians can develop more sophisticated assessment approaches that address the full range of presentations encountered in adult autism assessment.

Case 1 involves a 19-year-old female university student with depression, anxiety, and high academic achievement who was referred for autism assessment after struggling with the transition to university life. This case exemplifies several common assessment challenges, particularly related to female presentation, comorbid mental health conditions, and high cognitive abilities masking developmental differences.

The presentation includes several elements requiring careful assessment consideration.

The 19-year-old female university student presented with a complex clinical picture includes:

1. Long-standing depression and anxiety that had been treated with both medication and psychological therapy since age 16, with partial response
2. Exceptional academic achievement throughout school, with particular strengths in mathematics and physics
3. Significant social difficulties that became more apparent after transitioning to university, including challenges making friends, understanding social norms in student accommodation, and navigating group work
4. Sensory sensitivities affecting daily functioning, particularly noise sensitivity in lecture halls and student social spaces
5. Intense interest in astronomy that occupied much of her free time, with extensive knowledge beyond her university coursework

This presentation combines strengths in specific cognitive domains with challenges in social adaptation and emotional regulation, creating a complex clinical picture requiring careful assessment to distinguish between autism, mental health conditions, and typical adjustment difficulties.

Challenges in this assessment include several factors that complicate straightforward application of standard assessment approaches.

Strong camouflaging represents a significant assessment challenge in this case. The young woman demonstrated sophisticated strategies for masking social communication differences, including:

1. Careful observation and imitation of peer behaviour in social settings
2. Preparation of conversation topics and questions before social interactions
3. Conscious monitoring of facial expression and eye contact during conversation
4. Strategic use of her academic strengths to create social connections through study groups
5. Retreat to "bathroom breaks" when feeling overwhelmed, allowing private recovery before returning to social situations

These camouflaging strategies made her autism features less immediately apparent in structured assessment settings, requiring specific approaches to identify the underlying social communication differences and their impact.

High verbal abilities effectively masked some social difficulties, as her excellent vocabulary, grammar, and verbal reasoning created an initial impression of strong communication skills. However, careful assessment revealed:

1. Difficulties with the pragmatic aspects of language despite strong structural language
2. Literal interpretation of idioms and figures of speech despite understanding their meaning when explicitly questioned
3. Formal, pedantic speech style that stood out from typical peer communication
4. Challenges with conversational turn-taking, including difficulty identifying appropriate times to contribute
5. Limited modulation of verbal communication based on the social context or listener needs

These subtle pragmatic language differences required assessment approaches sensitive to the distinction between vocabulary and grammar versus social use of language.

Complex mental health presentation created diagnostic complexity, as many features could potentially be attributed to either autism or mental health conditions. Her anxiety and depression manifested in:

1. Social withdrawal that could reflect either social anxiety or autism-related social communication challenges
2. Repetitive behaviour's that might represent either autism features or anxiety compulsions
3. Sensory sensitivities that could be interpreted as either autism-related or anxiety-heightened sensory processing
4. Emotional dysregulation that might reflect either mood disorder or autism with co-occurring emotional challenges
5. Special interest intensity that could be viewed as either an autism feature or a coping mechanism for depression

Disentangling these overlapping presentations required careful developmental assessment and exploration of the temporal relationship between different symptoms.

The assessment approach for this complex case required specific adaptations to identify autism features that might be masked by compensatory strategies, gender-specific presentation, and mental health conditions.

Detailed developmental history from parents was particularly valuable in this case, as it revealed early indicators of autism that had been interpreted differently at the time:

1. Early preference for solitary play alongside rather than with other children
2. Intense childhood interests in collecting and categorizing rocks and minerals
3. Distress with changes in routine that had been attributed to "being particular"
4. Early sensory sensitivities to clothing textures, food consistencies, and noisy environments
5. Sophisticated vocabulary and reading skills developing earlier than social understanding

This developmental perspective provided crucial evidence of longstanding neurodevelopmental differences despite current compensatory strategies.

Exploration of social understanding versus social performance revealed a significant discrepancy between intellectual knowledge about social rules and intuitive social understanding:

1. Ability to explain social rules explicitly when asked, but difficulty applying them in real-time social situations
2. Recognition of her own social challenges with insight into specific difficulties
3. Description of social interaction as mentally exhausting due to constant conscious monitoring and analysis
4. Reports of "getting it wrong" despite careful attention to social cues
5. Explicit learning of social behaviour through observation, analysis, and practice rather than intuitive acquisition

This exploration highlighted the effortful, cognitive approach to social interaction characteristic of many autistic individuals with strong compensatory strategies.

Assessment in multiple contexts provided important information about how presentation varied across different environments and demands:

1. More apparent autism features during unstructured components of the assessment compared to structured interviews
2. Increasing stimming behaviour's (hair twirling, finger rubbing) as assessment sessions progressed and energy for compensation diminished
3. Greater social communication differences when discussing emotional rather than factual topics
4. Parental reports of significantly more obvious autism features at home after school throughout childhood ("holding it together" at school then "melting down" at home)
5. University observations of difficulties in informal social settings despite appropriate behaviour in lecture and seminar contexts

This contextual assessment revealed how compensatory strategies varied across settings and with different levels of fatigue or stress.

Focus on sensory and special interest patterns provided additional diagnostic information less affected by camouflaging:

1. Detailed assessment of sensory processing across multiple domains, revealing specific patterns of hyper- and hyposensitivity
2. Exploration of her astronomical interest, which demonstrated the intensity, systematic approach, and immersive quality characteristic of autism special interests
3. Assessment of sensory seeking behaviour's that became more apparent during periods of stress

4. Examination of routines and rituals related to managing sensory environment
5. Discussion of how sensory experiences affected participation in university activities

These aspects of the restricted and repetitive behaviour domain often show less gender-based variation than social communication features, providing important diagnostic information when female social camouflaging is present.

The outcome of this comprehensive assessment process was an autism diagnosis with specific recommendations for university accommodations:

Diagnostic conclusion was reached based on the integration of multiple information sources, which collectively indicated that despite strong compensatory strategies, the underlying pattern of social communication differences and restricted, repetitive behaviour was consistent with autism spectrum disorder. The formulation recognized both the clarity of autism features in early development and the increasingly sophisticated camouflaging that had developed over time.

Specific recommendations for university support included:

1. Sensory accommodations including permission to wear noise-cancelling headphones in lectures and priority housing in quieter residential areas
2. Academic adjustments including advance provision of changes to schedules or assignments and alternative arrangements for group work
3. Access to a mentor with autism expertise to provide support with social interpretation and university navigation
4. Structured opportunities for social connection based on shared interests
5. Continued mental health support addressing co-occurring anxiety and depression, adapted with understanding of autism context

These targeted recommendations addressed the specific challenges identified during assessment while building on her considerable strengths and existing coping strategies.

Education about female autism presentation was provided both to the young woman herself and, with her permission, to her parents and university disability service. This education included:

1. Information about how autism may present differently in females, particularly regarding social camouflaging
2. Explanation of the relationship between camouflaging effort and subsequent exhaustion

3. Recognition of her longstanding coping strategies and their effectiveness in many contexts
4. Discussion of how autism relates to her specific strengths and challenges
5. Guidance on selective disclosure decisions in different university contexts

This educational component supported positive identity development and enhanced self-advocacy skills within the university environment.

This case illustrates several important assessment principles for similar complex presentations:

1. The critical importance of developmental history when current presentation is complicated by compensatory strategies
2. The need for assessment approaches sensitive to female autism presentation, particularly regarding social camouflaging
3. The value of observing behaviour across different contexts and as compensation fatigue occurs
4. The importance of distinguishing between social knowledge and intuitive social understanding
5. The recognition that high academic achievement and strong verbal abilities can mask significant autism features
6. The need for recommendations that address both autism-specific needs and co-occurring mental health conditions

By applying these principles to similar complex presentations, clinicians can conduct more accurate assessments of individuals whose autism features might otherwise be missed due to gender, compensation, or mental health considerations.

CHAPTER 39

Complex Case Examples - Case 2

Case 2 involves a 45-year-old male with a history of employment difficulties, multiple job losses, and relationship breakdown who self-referred for autism assessment after reading about autism in adults and recognizing similarities with his own experiences. This case exemplifies the challenges of assessing older adults with limited developmental information, complex life histories, and multiple potentially overlapping conditions.

The presentation includes several elements requiring careful assessment consideration.

The 45-year-old male presented with a long history of occupational and relationship difficulties:

1. Pattern of securing jobs based on strong technical skills but losing them due to "personality conflicts," misunderstanding expectations, or difficulty adapting to workplace changes
2. History of three failed long-term relationships, with partners describing him as emotionally distant, rigid in routines, and difficult to connect with
3. Strong circumscribed interests in computer programming and medieval history, with exceptional knowledge in these areas
4. Sensory sensitivities affecting daily functioning, particularly to certain clothing textures, food consistencies, and background noise
5. Difficulties with executive functioning, including time management, organization, and task prioritization
6. History of anxiety and episodes of depression, with multiple brief courses of psychological therapy with limited benefit

This presentation combines specific areas of strength with persistent difficulties across occupational and relationship domains spanning several decades, suggesting longstanding differences rather than recent-onset difficulties.

Challenges in this assessment include several factors that complicate straightforward application of standard assessment approaches.

Limited developmental information presented a significant challenge, as the individual's parents were deceased, and he had no siblings or other family members who knew him during childhood. Available developmental information was limited to:

1. The individual's own recollections of childhood, which were somewhat vague and limited regarding social development
2. A few school reports from secondary education noting academic strengths alongside "difficulties working cooperatively" and being "somewhat inflexible"
3. No available records from primary education or early development
4. No informants with knowledge of his childhood social communication or behaviour patterns
5. Limited photographic or video records from childhood

This sparse developmental information made it difficult to establish the developmental history essential for autism diagnosis, requiring alternative approaches to determining whether current features reflected lifelong patterns.

Co-occurring ADHD and anxiety created diagnostic complexity, as the individual also displayed features consistent with these conditions, including:

1. Difficulties with sustained attention, organization, and time management suggestive of ADHD
2. Significant anxiety in social situations with worry about negative evaluation
3. Restlessness and difficulty sitting still during assessment
4. Perfectionism and fear of making mistakes potentially reflecting anxiety
5. Difficulty separating anxiety symptoms from social communication challenges

Disentangling these overlapping presentations required careful assessment of the timing, context, and quality of different symptoms to determine their relationship to potential autism.

Long history of compensating strategies had developed over decades of trying to navigate social and occupational demands, including:

1. Scripted responses for common social situations
2. Explicit study of facial expressions and their meanings
3. Careful observation and imitation of colleagues' social behaviour

4. Strategic use of technical expertise to create value in workplace settings despite social difficulties
5. Development of structured routines to compensate for executive functioning challenges

These compensatory strategies, developed over many years, made current autism features presently less obvious in some contexts, requiring assessment approaches that could identify underlying differences despite these adaptations.

The assessment approach for this complex case required specific adaptations to address the limited developmental information, complex clinical presentation, and longstanding compensatory strategies.

Extended self-report history focused on establishing patterns across the lifespan through detailed exploration of experiences in different life periods:

1. Structured timeline approach mapping social, occupational, and relationship experiences from earliest memories to present
2. Focused questioning about specific autism-related features in each life period
3. Exploration of subjective experiences in social situations throughout life
4. Detailed discussion of special interests, sensory experiences, and routines across different life stages
5. Comparison of experiences across different contexts (education, employment, relationships) to identify consistent patterns

This extended historical approach helped establish whether current features reflected longstanding patterns consistent with a developmental condition rather than acquired characteristics.

Workplace observational information was sought to supplement direct assessment:

1. With consent, obtaining detailed feedback from current employer about social communication and behavioural patterns in the workplace
2. Review of performance evaluations from previous employment when available
3. Discussion with an occupational health professional who had observed the individual in work contexts
4. Completion of structured questionnaires by current work supervisor regarding social communication and flexibility
5. Exploration of specific workplace incidents that illustrated social communication difficulties or restricted/repetitive behaviour

This collateral information from occupational contexts provided valuable observational data that compensated somewhat for the limited developmental information from childhood.

Standardized assessments were used with careful interpretation considering the limited normative data for older adults:

1. Administration of the **ADOS-2 Module 4**, with attention to qualitative aspects of performance beyond scoring algorithms
2. **Autism Spectrum Quotient (AQ)** and other self-report measures, considered in context of potential limited self-awareness
3. **Conners' Adult ADHD Rating Scales** to assess attention and hyperactivity symptoms
4. Assessments of **executive functioning**, including both standardized tests and functional measures
5. Anxiety measures to clarify the extent and nature of anxiety symptoms

These standardized measures provided structured assessment data while recognizing the limitations of instruments primarily validated with younger populations.

Trial interventions approach was implemented when diagnostic certainty remained limited after initial assessment:

1. Implementation of specific autism-informed strategies for workplace communication and organization
2. Environmental modifications addressing sensory sensitivities
3. Explicit social communication guidance using autism-specific approaches
4. Introduction of structured routines to support executive functioning
5. Monitoring response to these autism-specific interventions over a three-month period

This trial interventions approach provided additional diagnostic information through observation of response to autism-specific supports, which showed significant benefit suggesting good fit between autism-informed approaches and the individual's needs.

The outcome of this comprehensive assessment process was a provisional autism diagnosis with recommended supports:

Diagnostic conclusion involved provisional autism spectrum disorder diagnosis based on:

1. Current presentation consistent with autism features across social communication and restricted/repetitive behaviour domains
2. Evidence of longstanding patterns of difference from self-report history and available records
3. Exclusion of alternative explanations that could better account for the presenting features
4. Positive response to autism-specific interventions during the trial period
5. Consensus among the assessment team that autism best explained the overall clinical picture

The provisional nature of the diagnosis acknowledged the limitations in developmental history while recognizing the strong evidence from current functioning and historical patterns.

Comorbid condition assessment identified co-occurring ADHD and anxiety:

1. Attention and executive functioning difficulties exceeding typical autism-related challenges
2. Clear anxiety symptoms that exacerbated but did not fully explain social difficulties
3. Recommendation for specific ADHD assessment and potential medication trial
4. Anxiety management recommendations adapted for autism context
5. Recognition of how these conditions interacted with and amplified autism features

This comprehensive diagnostic formulation addressed the full clinical complexity rather than attempting to attribute all features to a single condition.

Support recommendations were practical and specific:

1. Workplace accommodations addressing both autism and ADHD-related needs
2. Structured approaches to relationship building based on autism-informed strategies
3. Environmental modifications for sensory sensitivities
4. Technology-based supports for executive functioning challenges
5. Connection with autism peer support for adults diagnosed later in life

These recommendations directly addressed the functional challenges that had prompted assessment while building on identified strengths and existing coping strategies.

Post-diagnostic therapy focusing on understanding and adapting to the diagnosis in mid-life:

1. Psychoeducation about autism and its manifestation in his specific case
2. Reframing of past experiences through the lens of autism understanding
3. Development of greater self-awareness and self-advocacy skills
4. Strategies for disclosure decisions in different contexts
5. Approaches for building more satisfying relationships with autism-informed communication strategies

This therapeutic support addressed the psychological impact of receiving a significant diagnosis in mid-life and provided practical strategies for moving forward with this new understanding.

This case illustrates several important assessment principles for similar complex presentations:

1. The challenge of establishing developmental history when conventional informants are unavailable
2. The importance of identifying patterns across different life domains and periods when childhood information is limited
3. The value of collateral information from workplace or other current contexts when developmental informants are unavailable
4. The potential utility of trial interventions as an additional source of diagnostic information in uncertain cases
5. The need to assess and address co-occurring conditions as part of comprehensive formulation

CHAPTER 40

Research Updates in Adult ASD

Staying current with research developments in adult autism is essential for evidence-based assessment practice. Recent years have seen significant advances in understanding adult autism presentations, developing assessment approaches, and identifying neurobiological markers. These research developments continue to refine and sometimes challenge established clinical practices, highlighting the evolving nature of our understanding of autism across the lifespan. Awareness of current research trends helps clinicians incorporate emerging knowledge into assessment approaches while maintaining appropriate scientific caution about preliminary findings.

Emerging assessment approaches reflect ongoing efforts to develop more sensitive, specific, and clinically useful tools for adult autism assessment.

Digital phenotyping represents an innovative approach using technology to capture behavioural data relevant to autism diagnosis. These approaches include:

1. Smartphone-based passive monitoring of social interaction patterns, activity levels, and daily routines
2. Computer vision analysis of facial expressions, eye movements, and nonverbal behaviour's during social interaction
3. Natural language processing examining linguistic patterns in speech or written communication
4. Virtual reality social scenarios providing standardized social challenges with precise measurement
5. Wearable sensors tracking physiological responses to social and sensory stimuli

These digital approaches offer potential advantages of objective measurement, continuous data collection in natural environments, and quantification of subtle behavioural differences that might be missed in traditional clinical observation. While most remain primarily research tools, some are beginning to enter clinical practice as supplementary assessment methods.

Biomarkers research explores potential biological indicators of autism that might support more objective diagnosis. Areas of investigation include:

1. Genetic markers, including both rare variants with large effects and common variants with smaller contributions
2. Epigenetic patterns that might reflect gene-environment interactions
3. Proteomic and metabolomic profiles in blood or other tissues
4. Immune and inflammatory markers that might indicate neuroinflammatory processes
5. Gut microbiome composition reflecting emerging understanding of gut-brain connections

While these biomarker approaches show promise for enhancing understanding of autism mechanisms, they remain primarily research tools with limited current clinical application. The heterogeneity of autism presents particular challenges for biomarker development, as different biological pathways may contribute to similar clinical presentations.

Neuroimaging correlates of autism are being investigated using various brain imaging techniques to identify structural and functional differences associated with autism. Research approaches include:

1. Functional MRI examining brain activation patterns during social cognition, language processing, and other relevant tasks
2. Structural MRI assessing differences in grey matter volume, cortical thickness, and white matter integrity
3. Diffusion tensor imaging investigating connectivity between brain regions
4. Magnetic resonance spectroscopy measuring neurochemical profiles
5. Electroencephalography and magnetoencephalography examining temporal dynamics of brain activity

These neuroimaging studies have identified group-level differences between autistic and non-autistic individuals, but considerable overlap and heterogeneity limit current clinical applications for individual diagnosis. Research increasingly focuses on identifying distinct neurobiological subtypes within the autism spectrum rather than seeking universal biomarkers.

Adult-specific measures are being developed and validated to address limitations of existing instruments primarily designed for children:

1. New self-report measures specifically designed for adults with autism, incorporating their lived experience in item development

2. Observational assessments appropriate for adult social contexts rather than play-based child scenarios
3. Measures sensitive to female autism presentation and camouflaging
4. Instruments validated across diverse cultural contexts to reduce cultural bias
5. Assessment tools specifically designed for adults with intellectual disabilities

These adult-specific measures aim to increase diagnostic accuracy by better capturing the unique manifestations of autism in adulthood, which may differ qualitatively from childhood presentations due to development, adaptation, and compensation.

Female presentation research has expanded significantly, providing more nuanced understanding of gender differences in autism:

Growing research base on female autism presentations has identified several key differences that impact assessment:

1. More sophisticated social camouflaging strategies in females, including careful observation and imitation of socially successful peers
2. Different manifestations of restricted interests that may appear more socially acceptable (e.g., interests in literature, psychology, or animals rather than technical systems)
3. Different presentation of repetitive behaviour's, with fewer obvious motor stereotypies and more subtle repetitive patterns
4. Stronger language and social imitation skills potentially masking underlying social understanding differences
5. Greater vulnerability to internalizing conditions such as anxiety and depression that may obscure underlying autism

This research highlights the need for gender-informed assessment approaches that account for these qualitative differences in presentation, potentially including different thresholds or modified criteria for females.

Research on camouflaging has evolved from clinical observation to systematic investigation, examining:

1. Mechanisms of camouflaging, including both conscious strategies and unconscious adaptations
2. Measurement approaches to quantify camouflaging, such as discrepancy between external presentation and internal experience

3. Negative impacts of camouflaging on mental health, including links to anxiety, depression, and suicidality
4. Differences in camouflaging across gender, age, and cultural groups
5. Neurobiological correlates of camouflaging ability and effort

This research provides empirical support for clinical observations about compensation strategies and helps develop more sensitive approaches to identifying autism despite effective camouflaging.

Intersectional factors research examines how autism interacts with other aspects of identity and experience:

1. Cultural influences on autism expression, recognition, and impact
2. Socioeconomic factors affecting access to diagnosis and support
3. Gender identity and sexual orientation diversity in the autism population
4. Racial and ethnic disparities in autism identification and service access
5. Interaction between autism and trauma experiences

This intersectional research highlights the need for assessment approaches that consider multiple dimensions of identity and experience rather than viewing autism in isolation from other aspects of the individual's life and context.

Adult outcomes longitudinal studies provide valuable information about developmental trajectories and long-term outcomes.

Long-term follow-up studies of individuals diagnosed in childhood have examined outcomes across multiple domains:

1. Significant heterogeneity in adult outcomes, ranging from independent living and employment to ongoing high support needs
2. Identification of childhood predictors of adult outcomes, including early language development and cognitive abilities
3. Common challenges in educational attainment, employment, independent living, and relationship development
4. Impact of appropriate support on improving outcomes across domains
5. Persistence of autism features throughout adulthood with some changes in manifestation

These longitudinal findings highlight both the stability of core autism features across the lifespan and the potential for positive development and adaptation with appropriate support.

Quality of life research has expanded beyond functional outcomes to examine subjective well-being and life satisfaction:

1. Identification of factors contributing to quality of life in autistic adults, including sense of belonging, autonomy, and acceptance
2. Development of autism-specific quality of life measures that capture domains particularly relevant to autistic experience
3. Growing evidence that acceptance and accommodation may contribute more to well-being than symptom reduction
4. Recognition of the impact of co-occurring conditions, particularly anxiety and depression, on quality of life
5. Exploration of autistic perspectives on what constitutes a good life, which may differ from normative assumptions

This quality-of-life research enriches outcome measurement beyond traditional functional indicators to include subjective well-being and life satisfaction from autistic perspectives.

UK research centres leading studies in adult autism include several institutions with specialized expertise:

University of Cambridge Autism Research Centre, led by **Professor Simon Baron-Cohen**, focuses on:

1. Cognitive and neuroscience studies of autism across the lifespan
2. Development and validation of screening and diagnostic instruments
3. Investigation of potential biological markers
4. Research on female autism presentation
5. Employment support models for autistic adults

King's College London Institute of Psychiatry, Psychology & Neuroscience conducts research on:

1. Adult autism diagnosis and support
2. Transition from child to adult services
3. Co-occurring mental health conditions
4. Neuroimaging studies of autism
5. Longitudinal outcomes in adulthood

Newcastle University conducts significant adult autism research focusing on:

1. Autism in older adults
2. Adult diagnostic pathways

3. Gender differences in autism presentation
4. Mental health in autistic adults
5. Service design and implementation

University College London Centre for Research in Autism and Education emphasizes:

1. Participatory research methods involving autistic collaborators
2. Educational and employment outcomes
3. Development of support models
4. Sensory processing differences
5. Gender diversity in the autism population

These UK research centres offer opportunities for clinicians to engage with cutting-edge research through conferences, publications, training events, and potential research participation.

Clinical implications of research findings for assessment practice include several important considerations:

Translating research to practice requires thoughtful consideration of which findings are sufficiently established to inform clinical approaches. Key translation principles include:

1. Distinguishing between well-established findings with multiple replications and preliminary results requiring further validation
2. Considering both statistical significance and clinical significance when evaluating research findings
3. Recognizing limitations of study samples and methods when generalizing to clinical populations
4. Balancing innovation with ethical responsibility to use established approaches
5. Involving autistic perspectives in determining how research should inform practice

These principles support responsible integration of research advances into clinical practice while maintaining appropriate scientific caution.

Emerging assessment recommendations based on current research include:

1. Greater attention to camouflaging and compensation strategies, particularly when assessing females and adults with higher cognitive abilities

2. Consideration of sensory differences as a core feature rather than a secondary aspect of autism
3. Recognition of executive functioning challenges as common in autism and relevant to functional impact
4. Inclusion of autistic perspectives in the assessment process through partnership approaches
5. Consideration of quality of life and well-being outcomes rather than focusing exclusively on symptom reduction

These emerging recommendations reflect evolving understanding of autism features and assessment approaches based on recent research developments.

Future directions in adult autism assessment research include several promising areas:

1. Development of telehealth assessment models that combine remote and in-person components for greater accessibility
2. Creation and validation of more culturally diverse assessment measures and approaches
3. Integration of objective digital measurements with clinical judgment
4. Refinement of assessment approaches for complex or atypical presentations
5. Implementation research examining how to effectively translate research advances into clinical practice across diverse service settings

These future directions highlight the dynamic nature of autism assessment, with ongoing development and refinement of approaches based on evolving research evidence.

By maintaining awareness of current research developments while applying appropriate critical evaluation, clinicians can ensure that assessment practices reflect contemporary understanding of adult autism while maintaining necessary scientific rigor.

CHAPTER 41
Training and Supervision Requirements

Effective autism assessment requires specific training and ongoing supervision to ensure high-quality, evidence-based practice. The complexity of autism presentation, the evolving nature of assessment approaches, and the significant implications of diagnostic decisions necessitate both initial specialized training and continuing professional development. Understanding the training and supervision requirements for autism assessment helps ensure that clinicians develop and maintain the specialized skills needed for this challenging clinical area.

ADOS-2 and **ADI-R** formal certification requirements represent essential training for clinicians conducting comprehensive autism assessments:

Formal certification for the ADOS-2 is mandatory for valid administration and interpretation. This certification typically involves:

1. Attendance at a 2 to3 days of clinical training workshop led by certified trainers
2. Detailed instruction in administration procedures, scoring conventions, and diagnostic algorithms
3. Practice scoring of standardized video recordings to establish reliability
4. Supervised practice administrations following the workshop
5. Demonstration of scoring reliability compared to established standards

This rigorous training process ensures standardized administration and interpretation, which is essential for maintaining the psychometric properties of the instrument. Use of the ADOS-2 without this formal training compromises the validity of results and would not meet professional standards for evidence-based assessment.

Formal certification for the ADI-R follows a similar process, including:

1. Attendance at a 2 to3 days of specialized training workshop

2. Instruction in interview techniques, coding conventions, and algorithm application
3. Practice coding of standardized interview recordings
4. Supervised practice administrations
5. Reliability establishment through comparison with expert coding

This formal training is essential for valid administration of this complex developmental interview, ensuring standardized gathering and interpretation of historical information crucial for autism diagnosis.

UK training providers for these essential instruments include:

Pearson Assessment, **the UK distributor for the ADOS-2 and ADI-R**, offers regular training workshops in various locations throughout the UK. These training events provide the formal certification required for clinical use of these instruments and often include options for establishing research reliability for those conducting research studies.

University College London (UCL) regularly hosts ADOS-2 and ADI-R training through its clinical psychology and psychiatry departments. These trainings often include opportunities for observation of expert administration and follow-up supervision to support implementation in clinical practice.

University of Manchester Social Development Research Group provides specialized training in both instruments with particular expertise in complex presentations and cultural considerations. Their training programs emphasize clinical application in diverse populations.

Newcastle University Autism Research Centre offers periodic training with a focus on adult assessment applications, particularly addressing the challenges of using these instruments with adults without intellectual disabilities and those with complex or atypical presentations.

The National Autistic Society occasionally partners with clinical experts to provide training in these instruments, often incorporating perspectives from autistic individuals to enhance understanding of the lived experience behind the behaviour's being assessed.

Maintenance of reliability after initial certification requires ongoing attention to preserve assessment quality:

Regular practice is essential for maintaining skills, with recommendations of:

1. Conducting at least one ADOS-2 or ADI-R administration monthly to maintain procedural fluency
2. Regular scoring review with colleagues to prevent drift from standardized coding conventions
3. Periodic video review of administrations to monitor adherence to standardized procedures
4. Annual review of manual sections covering challenging or infrequently encountered scoring decisions
5. Implementation of structured quality checks for consistency across time

Regular participation in consensus coding meetings, where team members independently score the same administration and then discuss discrepancies, provides valuable ongoing calibration of scoring judgments and prevents idiosyncratic interpretation.

Refresh training is recommended every 2-3 years, particularly when:

1. Clinical responsibilities have limited regular use of the instruments
2. New versions or updates to the instruments have been released
3. Expanding use to different populations (e.g., from children to adults)
4. Assessment practices have drifted from standardized procedures
5. New team members need orientation to team-based implementation

This ongoing attention to reliability maintenance ensures that the initial investment in training continues to support valid assessment over time.

Clinical supervision represents an essential component of quality assurance in autism assessment:

Recommended supervision structure for clinicians conducting autism assessments includes:

1. Regular case-based supervision focusing on complex or challenging assessments
2. Periodic direct observation of assessment practice with feedback
3. Review of assessment reports to ensure comprehensive documentation and sound diagnostic reasoning
4. Team-based supervision allowing multiple perspectives on complex presentations

5. Access to more experienced clinicians for consultation on particularly challenging cases

For early-career clinicians or those new to autism assessment, more intensive supervision is appropriate, potentially including observation of all initial assessments and co-working arrangements until competence is established. As experience develops, supervision may shift toward focus on complex cases and quality assurance.

Supervision content should address various aspects of assessment practice:

1. Appropriate selection and adaptation of assessment methods for individual presentations
2. Interpretation of sometimes contradictory information from different sources
3. Distinction between autism and potential differential diagnoses
4. Cultural considerations in assessment and interpretation
5. Ethical issues in diagnostic decision-making
6. Communication of findings to individuals and families
7. Development of appropriate recommendations based on assessment findings

This comprehensive supervision ensures development of clinical judgment that extends beyond technical proficiency with assessment instruments to encompass the full complexity of autism assessment.

Regular case discussions with multi-disciplinary colleagues provide valuable opportunities for:

1. Integration of perspectives from different professional disciplines
2. Consideration of alternative interpretations of assessment findings
3. Identification of potential biases or assumptions affecting interpretation
4. Development of more comprehensive formulation and recommendations
5. Ongoing professional development through exposure to varied clinical perspectives

These case discussions are particularly valuable for complex or atypical presentations where standard assessment approaches may require adaptation or particularly careful interpretation.

Continuing professional development beyond formal instrument training is essential for maintaining and expanding assessment expertise:

Royal College requirements establish minimum standards for **continuing professional development (CPD)** that apply to autism assessment practice:

The Royal College of Psychiatrists requires members to complete a minimum of 50 hours of CPD annually, with activities relevant to their scope of practice. For psychiatrists involved in autism assessment, this should include specific activities focused on autism and neurodevelopmental conditions alongside broader psychiatric CPD.

The British Psychological Society similarly requires chartered psychologists to maintain regular CPD activities relevant to their practice areas, documented through their professional development logs. For psychologists conducting autism assessments, specialized neurodevelopmental CPD should form a core component of their overall professional development.

Other professional bodies including **the Royal College of Speech and Language Therapists, Royal College of Occupational Therapists, and Nursing and Midwifery Council** maintain similar requirements for ongoing professional development relevant to specific practice areas.

These professional requirements establish minimum standards, but comprehensive expertise in autism assessment typically requires more extensive and focused development activities.

Autism-specific training opportunities beyond basic instrument certification include:

Specialized workshops on specific aspects of autism assessment, such as:

1. Assessment of females with autism
2. Cultural considerations in autism diagnosis
3. Distinguishing autism from complex trauma presentations
4. Assessment of adults with intellectual disabilities
5. Identification of autism in the context of co-occurring mental health conditions

University-based certificate or diploma programs providing comprehensive training in autism assessment and support, such as those offered by:

1. University College London's Postgraduate Certificate in Autism Spectrum Disorders
2. University of Birmingham's Autism Studies programs
3. Manchester Metropolitan University's Autism Spectrum Conditions courses

4. Queen's University Belfast's Applied Behaviour Analysis and Autism programs
5. Various online learning programs from UK universities focusing on autism assessment and support

These more extensive educational programs provide depth of understanding beyond what can be achieved through brief workshop formats.

Conferences focusing on adult autism provide valuable opportunities for learning about current research and clinical advances:

1. National Autistic Society Professional Conferences
2. Association for Psychological Therapies Autism Conferences
3. Autism Europe International Congress (held every three years)
4. International Society for Autism Research (INSAR) Annual Meeting
5. Various NHS and university-hosted specialist conferences

These events provide exposure to current research developments, innovative assessment approaches, and opportunities to network with other professionals with autism expertise.

Self-directed learning through various media supplements formal training:

1. Peer-reviewed journals focusing on autism research and practice
2. Professional books addressing specific aspects of autism assessment
3. Online learning modules from professional organizations
4. Webinars and video resources from expert clinicians
5. Podcasts featuring autism researchers and clinicians discussing current topics

This self-directed learning allows clinicians to focus on specific areas of interest or need within the broader field of autism assessment.

Lived experience input represents an increasingly recognized component of professional development:

Learning from autistic perspectives provides essential insights that complement traditional clinical training:

1. Training and presentations delivered by autistic professionals
2. Panels featuring autistic adults discussing their diagnostic experiences
3. Collaborative learning events bringing together autistic individuals and clinicians
4. Autistic-authored books, blogs, and other media sharing lived experience

5. Partnerships with autistic consultants in service development and evaluation

This lived experience input helps clinicians understand the subjective experience behind the behaviours and differences they observe in clinical assessment, potentially enhancing both accuracy and sensitivity in the assessment process.

Formal inclusion of autistic trainers in professional education has increased, with many training programs now incorporating:

1. Co-facilitation of workshops by autistic and non-autistic trainers
2. Development of training materials in partnership with autistic consultants
3. Evaluation of training effectiveness from both clinical and autistic perspectives
4. Mentoring relationships between autistic adults and clinicians developing assessment skills
5. Service user involvement in clinical supervision discussions

This collaborative approach to professional development recognizes the complementary expertise that autistic perspectives bring to clinical training.

Online learning opportunities have expanded significantly, particularly since the COVID-19 pandemic, providing:

1. Greater accessibility for clinicians in geographically remote areas
2. Flexibility for integrating professional development with clinical responsibilities
3. Opportunities to learn from international experts without travel requirements
4. Recorded content that can be reviewed multiple times for deeper learning
5. Interactive formats allowing for question-and-answer engagement with experts

These online options significantly expand access to specialized training that might previously have been limited by geographic or resource constraints.

Multi-disciplinary learning initiatives bring together professionals from different disciplines involved in autism assessment:

Joint training across disciplines offers valuable opportunities for:

1. Understanding different professional perspectives on autism assessment
2. Developing common language and conceptual frameworks across disciplines

3. Building collaborative relationships that support integrated assessment approaches
4. Learning assessment techniques and perspectives from complementary professional traditions
5. Creating more cohesive multi-disciplinary assessment teams through shared learning experiences

These multi-disciplinary learning opportunities reflect the inherently multi-disciplinary nature of comprehensive autism assessment, which benefits from integration of diverse professional perspectives.

By meeting these training and supervision requirements, clinicians develop and maintain the specialized skills necessary for high-quality autism assessment. This professional development pathway combines formal instrument training, regular clinical supervision, continuing education, and integration of lived experience perspectives to build comprehensive assessment expertise.

CHAPTER 42

Quality Assurance in ASD Assessment

Quality assurance in autism assessment involves systematic approaches to ensuring consistent, accurate, and effective assessment practices across clinicians and over time. These quality measures help maintain high standards, identify areas for improvement, and demonstrate service effectiveness to commissioners and regulators. Implementing structured quality assurance processes benefits individuals being assessed by ensuring they receive accurate diagnosis and appropriate recommendations regardless of which clinician conducts their assessment or when it occurs.

Audit measures provide objective evaluation of assessment quality through systematic review of various aspects of the assessment process:

Diagnostic consistency represents a key quality indicator, examining the reliability of diagnostic decisions across different clinicians and cases. Audit approaches include:

1. Regular review of diagnostic rates across different clinicians within the same service, investigating patterns of significant variation
2. Second-clinician review of a random sample of assessments to evaluate consistency of diagnostic decisions
3. Comparison of diagnostic rates with epidemiological expectations and rates in comparable services
4. Follow-up assessment of a sample of cases to evaluate diagnostic stability over time
5. Analysis of patterns in diagnostic decision-making to identify potential biases related to demographic factors

These consistency audits help identify whether diagnostic thresholds are being applied uniformly and appropriately across the service, supporting both individual clinician development and service-wide quality improvement.

Report quality evaluation ensures that assessment documentation meets professional standards and effectively communicates findings. Audit methods include:

1. Structured review of reports against standardized quality criteria
2. Peer review of reports with feedback on strengths and areas for improvement
3. Evaluation of clarity, comprehensiveness, and accessibility of language
4. Assessment of how effectively reports translate findings into practical recommendations
5. Review of consistency between assessment data and diagnostic conclusions

These documentation audits help maintain high standards of clinical communication and ensure that reports serve their multiple purposes of justifying diagnostic decisions, providing useful understanding, and guiding subsequent support.

Service user satisfaction measurement provides crucial feedback about the assessment experience from those being assessed. Approaches include:

1. Post-assessment satisfaction questionnaires addressing various aspects of the assessment process
2. Feedback interviews exploring the assessment experience in greater depth
3. Focus groups with recently assessed individuals to identify common themes in experiences
4. Monitoring of complaints and compliments to identify patterns
5. Involvement of service users in designing quality measures that reflect their priorities

This service user perspective ensures that quality assurance addresses not only technical accuracy but also the subjective experience of assessment, which significantly impacts how diagnostic information is received and used.

Time standards monitoring evaluates the efficiency and timeliness of the assessment process. Audit measures include:

1. Waiting time from referral to first assessment appointment
2. Duration of the assessment process from first appointment to diagnostic decision
3. Time from diagnostic decision to report completion

4. Comparison of actual timeframes with service standards and national guidance
5. Analysis of factors contributing to delays in the assessment pathway

These efficiency measures help identify bottlenecks in the assessment process and ensure that individuals receive timely assessment without unnecessary delays that might prolong uncertainty or postpone access to appropriate support.

Peer review processes provide structured approaches to maintaining and improving assessment quality through collegial feedback and discussion:

Case discussion with different team members examining challenging or complex cases offers opportunities for:

1. Integration of multiple professional perspectives on diagnostic questions
2. Identification of additional assessment information that might clarify diagnostic uncertainty
3. Reflection on potential biases affecting diagnostic reasoning
4. Consideration of alternative interpretations of assessment findings
5. Development of more comprehensive formulation and recommendations

These case discussions enhance diagnostic accuracy through collective wisdom while also serving as valuable professional development for all participants.

Observation of assessment practice by experienced colleagues provides direct feedback on clinical skills:

1. Periodic observation of assessment sessions with subsequent reflective discussion
2. Co-working arrangements where two clinicians jointly conduct assessment components
3. Video recording of assessments (with consent) for later review and feedback
4. Structured feedback focusing on specific aspects of assessment technique
5. Identification of both strengths and development areas in assessment practice

This direct observation allows for coaching and skill development that cannot be achieved through case discussion alone, as it addresses not just diagnostic reasoning but the practical implementation of assessment approaches.

External peer review involving clinicians from other services provides valuable perspective:

1. Reciprocal arrangements between services for periodic review of assessment practices
2. External expert review of a sample of complex cases
3. Participation in regional clinical networks focused on autism assessment
4. Cross-service consensus coding sessions using video-recorded assessments
5. Collaborative audit projects examining assessment quality across multiple services

This external perspective helps prevent the development of service-specific practices that may drift from broader professional standards and provides fresh insights from different clinical contexts.

Regular clinical supervision structured to address quality as well as professional development ensures ongoing attention to assessment standards:

Regular individual supervision provides opportunities for:

1. Discussion of challenging cases and diagnostic dilemmas
2. Reflection on patterns in assessment practice and potential biases
3. Review of feedback from peer review and audit processes
4. Planning of professional development to address identified learning needs
5. Support for managing the emotional demands of complex assessment work

Group supervision sessions allow for:

1. Shared learning across the assessment team
2. Calibration of diagnostic thresholds through case examples
3. Discussion of service-wide quality issues and improvement approaches
4. Implementation of new evidence or guidelines across the whole team
5. Development of consistent approaches to common assessment challenges

This supervision infrastructure provides the foundation for maintaining individual and team quality standards while supporting ongoing professional development.

Service development based on quality findings creates a continuous improvement cycle:

Continuous improvement approaches systematically use quality information to enhance service delivery:

1. Regular review of quality data to identify patterns and trends
2. Root cause analysis of identified quality issues

3. Development of specific improvement initiatives addressing priority areas
4. PDSA (Plan-Do-Study-Act) cycles to test and refine improvement approaches
5. Re-audit following implementation to evaluate effectiveness of changes

This structured approach to service improvement ensures that quality assurance leads to concrete enhancements in assessment practice rather than simply measuring current performance.

Service user involvement in quality processes strengthens the relevance and effectiveness of improvement efforts:

1. Partnership with service users in designing quality measures and standards
2. Involvement of people with autism in reviewing and interpreting quality findings
3. Co-production of improvement initiatives with autistic consultants
4. Service user participation in governance structures overseeing quality
5. Employment of experts by experience in quality improvement roles

This collaborative approach ensures that quality standards reflect the priorities and perspectives of those being assessed rather than solely professional or organizational concerns.

Implementation science approaches apply evidence-based methods to translate research and guidelines into practice:

1. Systematic identification of barriers and facilitators to implementing best practices
2. Tailored implementation strategies addressing specific contextual factors
3. Measurement of both implementation outcomes (e.g., fidelity) and service outcomes
4. Attention to sustainability of practice changes beyond initial implementation
5. Organizational culture development supporting continuous evidence-based practice

These implementation science methods help bridge the gap between knowledge of best practices and their consistent application in routine clinical settings.

UK standards provide frameworks for quality assurance in autism assessment:

Adherence to national guidance forms a foundation for quality assurance, including:

NICE guidelines for autism assessment establish clear standards for comprehensive assessment, including:

1. Multi-disciplinary approach incorporating multiple perspectives
2. Detailed developmental history and current functioning assessment
3. Consideration of potential differential diagnoses
4. Structured discussion and consensus for diagnostic decision-making
5. Clear communication of findings and recommendations

Compliance with these evidence-based guidelines provides a baseline quality standard for all UK autism assessment services.

NHS England Autism Programme quality standards address system-level factors affecting assessment quality:

1. Specification of appropriate referral pathways and criteria
2. Standards for waiting times from referral to assessment
3. Requirements for professional training and supervision
4. Expectations for post-diagnostic support provision
5. Monitoring framework for service performance

These national standards provide benchmarks against which local services can evaluate their performance and identify improvement priorities.

Local clinical commissioning requirements often include specific quality standards tailored to local context:

1. Demographic-specific adaptations reflecting local population needs
2. Integration requirements with other local health and social care services
3. Specific outcome metrics reflecting local priorities
4. Reporting requirements for quality indicators
5. Service user involvement specifications for local implementation

Compliance with these commissioning requirements ensures that services meet local needs while maintaining national standards.

Professional standards from relevant bodies establish quality expectations for individual practitioners:

1. General Medical Council standards for medical practice
2. British Psychological Society professional practice guidelines

3. Royal College of Speech and Language Therapists clinical standards
4. Health and Care Professions Council standards of proficiency
5. Nursing and Midwifery Council Code of Practice

These professional standards complement service-level quality frameworks by establishing individual practitioner responsibilities for maintaining assessment quality.

Digital technologies increasingly support quality assurance in autism assessment:

Electronic health records facilitate systematic quality monitoring through:

1. Standardized documentation formats ensuring comprehensive assessment
2. Automated audit processes tracking key quality indicators
3. Decision support tools promoting evidence-based practice
4. Access to previous assessments supporting consistency over time
5. Integrated outcome measurement capturing impact of assessment and subsequent interventions

Assessment apps and digital tools provide structured approaches to gathering and integrating assessment information:

1. Tablet-based administration of standardized measures
2. Digital algorithms supporting diagnostic decision-making
3. Visualization tools displaying patterns across assessment components
4. Remote data collection expanding assessment beyond clinical settings
5. Video analysis tools enhancing observational assessment

These digital approaches enhance quality through structured processes, comprehensive data capture, and analytical capabilities that support more consistent and thorough assessment.

The benefits of robust quality assurance extend beyond regulatory compliance to fundamental improvements in assessment effectiveness:

Enhanced diagnostic accuracy benefits individuals through:

1. Appropriate identification of autism when present
2. Avoidance of misdiagnosis when other explanations better account for difficulties
3. Recognition of co-occurring conditions requiring specific interventions
4. Detailed understanding of individual strengths and challenges beyond diagnostic categories

5. Personalized recommendations based on comprehensive assessment

More effective support planning results from high-quality assessment through:

1. Clear identification of specific needs requiring support
2. Recognition of strengths that can be leveraged in intervention
3. Detailed understanding of environmental factors affecting functioning
4. Prioritization guidance for addressing multiple identified needs
5. Specific recommendations tailored to individual profile rather than generic approaches

Improved service user experience stems from quality-focused assessment:

1. Clear communication throughout the assessment process
2. Respectful, person-centred approaches to gathering information
3. Timely completion without unnecessary delays
4. Comprehensible explanation of findings and their implications
5. Meaningful involvement in support planning following assessment

By implementing comprehensive quality assurance processes, services can ensure that every individual receives assessment that meets these standards of accuracy, effectiveness, and positive experience, regardless of which clinician conducts their assessment or when it occurs in their journey.

CHAPTER 43

Common Pitfalls in Adult Assessment

Even experienced clinicians can encounter challenges in adult autism assessment that may compromise diagnostic accuracy or the effectiveness of the assessment process. Awareness of common pitfalls helps clinicians proactively avoid these issues or address them when they arise. Understanding these potential problems and their solutions supports more accurate, comprehensive, and helpful assessment for adults seeking autism evaluation.

Overlooking camouflaging represents one of the most significant pitfalls in adult assessment, particularly affecting diagnosis of females and individuals with higher cognitive abilities:

Failure to identify camouflaging strategies may lead to missed diagnoses when individuals have developed sophisticated approaches to masking their autism features in assessment situations. These strategies might include:

1. Careful preparation for social situations, including rehearsing responses and conversation topics
2. Deliberate management of eye contact, facial expression, and other nonverbal behaviour's
3. Imitation of others' social behaviours without intuitive understanding of their purpose
4. Strategic use of their intellectual strengths to compensate for social difficulties
5. Withdrawal to private spaces when overwhelmed to recover before continuing social engagement

Without specific assessment approaches to identify these camouflaging efforts, clinicians may observe apparently typical social behaviour while missing the underlying differences and significant effort required to produce this appearance of neurotypicality.

Identification approaches that help recognize camouflaging include:

1. Specific questioning about the subjective experience of social interaction, including mental effort, preparation, and aftermath
2. Extending assessment over multiple sessions to observe potential fatigue in maintaining camouflaging
3. Creating varied assessment contexts with different levels of structure and predictability
4. Gathering collateral information from those who know the individual in less formal contexts
5. Attending to discrepancies between self-report of difficulties and observed behaviour

These specialized approaches help penetrate the "social mask" that many adults with autism have developed, allowing for more accurate identification of underlying neurodevelopmental differences.

Particularly vulnerable groups who may be missed due to effective camouflaging include:

1. Females, who often develop more sophisticated social camouflaging strategies due to stronger social expectations and earlier feedback about social differences
2. Individuals with higher intellectual abilities who can apply their cognitive strengths to analysing and mimicking social behaviour
3. Those with strong language skills that mask underlying pragmatic language differences
4. Individuals from cultures with strong conformity expectations who have developed strict adherence to social rules
5. Those who have received prior social skills interventions that taught behavioural scripts without addressing underlying social cognition differences

Special attention to the possibility of camouflaging in these groups helps prevent diagnostic overshadowing by apparent social competence.

Overreliance on single measures creates significant risk of incomplete or biased assessment, as no single instrument captures the full complexity of adult autism presentation:

Limitations of specific instruments include:

1. The ADOS-2, while valuable for direct observation, may miss autism features in individuals with effective compensation strategies, particularly during brief, structured interactions
2. Self-report questionnaires depend on self-awareness and insight that may be limited in some individuals with autism
3. Developmental interviews like the ADI-R rely on informant memory and availability, which may be limited for older adults
4. Cognitive assessments may identify specific processing styles but don't directly assess core autism features
5. Screening tools designed for efficiency necessarily sacrifice comprehensiveness and may miss subtle presentations

These inherent limitations of individual measures necessitate multi-method assessment approaches that compensate for the weaknesses of any single instrument.

Comprehensive approaches that mitigate this pitfall include:

1. Integration of information from multiple sources, including standardized instruments, clinical interview, collateral reports, and historical documentation
2. Selection of complementary assessment methods that address different aspects of autism presentation
3. Consideration of convergence and divergence across different assessment components
4. Weighting of different information sources based on their reliability and relevance for the specific individual
5. Recognition that diagnostic decision-making requires clinical judgment informed by, but not determined solely by, standardized measures

This balanced, multi-method approach supports more accurate assessment than rigid adherence to cutoff scores or algorithms from any single instrument.

Diagnostic overshadowing involves attributing all features to one condition without recognizing potential co-occurring conditions or alternative explanations. This overshadowing can occur in several directions:

Missing ASD due to mental health presentation is common when prominent anxiety, depression, or other mental health symptoms mask underlying autism features. This may occur when:

1. Social withdrawal is attributed solely to depression rather than considering long-standing social communication differences
2. Social anxiety is identified without exploring whether it stems from actual difficulty understanding social rules rather than fear of negative evaluation
3. Emotional dysregulation is attributed to personality disorders without considering autism-related emotional processing differences
4. Obsessive-compulsive symptoms are diagnosed without recognizing the different quality and function of autism-related repetitive behaviour's
5. Attention difficulties are attributed solely to ADHD without considering the impact of autism-related sensory sensitivities or monotropic attention patterns

Careful developmental history and attention to the quality and context of symptoms helps distinguish between primary autism with secondary mental health conditions and primary mental health conditions without autism.

Similarly, attributing social difficulties to anxiety alone without considering underlying autism features represents a common oversight. Distinguishing factors include:

1. Whether social difficulties preceded anxiety or developed concurrently
2. The presence of social communication differences even in low-anxiety situations
3. Whether social understanding or merely social performance is affected
4. The presence of autism features beyond the social domain, such as restricted interests or sensory sensitivities
5. Response to anxiety-focused interventions—improvement in anxiety without corresponding improvement in social understanding suggests underlying autism

This careful differentiation between anxiety and autism features requires detailed developmental history and thoughtful exploration of the relationship between anxiety symptoms and social communication patterns.

Conversely, attributing all features to autism without recognizing co-occurring conditions represents another form of diagnostic overshadowing. Comprehensive assessment should consider:

1. Whether attention difficulties exceed what would be expected from autism alone
2. The presence of persistent low mood or anhedonia beyond situational responses

3. Anxiety symptoms that may warrant specific intervention beyond autism support
4. Possible co-occurring specific learning difficulties separate from autism features
5. Physical health conditions that may interact with and exacerbate autism features

Recognition of this complex interplay between autism and co-occurring conditions supports more comprehensive formulation and effective intervention planning.

Narrow developmental focus may lead to incomplete understanding of autism presentation across the lifespan:

Missing adult adaptations represents a significant risk when assessment focuses primarily on childhood manifestations of autism without recognizing how presentation evolves with development:

1. Social communication differences may become more subtle as individuals develop compensatory strategies and social scripts
2. Repetitive behaviours often become less overtly apparent as adults learn to manage or conceal them in public settings
3. Special interests may evolve toward more age-appropriate content while maintaining the same intensity and approach
4. Sensory sensitivities may be managed through environmental modifications and avoidance strategies
5. Executive functioning challenges may become more apparent as adult independence demands increase

Assessment approaches that focus narrowly on childhood manifestations without considering these developmental adaptations risk missing autism in adults who no longer present with the more obvious features typical in childhood.

Developmental assessment should examine patterns across the lifespan, including:

1. How social communication differences have manifested at different developmental stages
2. Evolution of restricted and repetitive behaviours from childhood to adulthood
3. Adaptation strategies developed over time and their effectiveness
4. Impact of life transitions on the manifestation of autism features

5. Current presentation in relation to developmental trajectory rather than in isolation

This lifespan perspective provides context for understanding current functioning as part of an ongoing developmental process rather than a static presentation.

Cultural misinterpretation creates risk of both false positive and false negative assessments when cultural differences are not adequately considered:

Misreading culturally-influenced behaviour's as autism features can occur when:

1. Cultural norms for eye contact differ from Western expectations
2. Culturally appropriate conversational styles involve different turn-taking or topic maintenance patterns
3. Culturally specific approaches to emotional expression are misinterpreted as restricted affect
4. Cultural practices involving routines or rituals are misunderstood as autism-related restricted behaviour's
5. Language differences or accents are mistaken for pragmatic language difficulties

These misinterpretations risk pathologizing cultural differences rather than accurately identifying neurodevelopmental variations.

Conversely, missing autism features due to cultural explanations represents the opposite risk, where genuine autism indicators are inappropriately attributed to cultural differences. This may occur when:

1. Genuine social communication difficulties beyond cultural norms are dismissed as merely cultural differences
2. Restricted and repetitive behaviours are incorrectly assumed to be culturally normative
3. Developmental concerns expressed differently across cultures are not recognized
4. Language differences mask underlying pragmatic language difficulties
5. Cultural factors affecting help-seeking or symptom reporting are not considered

These complex interactions between culture and autism presentation require sophisticated assessment approaches that can distinguish between cultural variations and autism features while recognizing their potential co-occurrence.

Culturally informed assessment approaches that mitigate these risks include:

1. Gathering specific information about the individual's cultural background and its behavioural norms
2. Consultation with cultural experts or interpreters beyond simple language translation
3. Comparison of behaviours to expectations within the individual's specific cultural context rather than Western norms
4. Adaptation of assessment methods and interpretation frameworks to accommodate cultural differences
5. Recognition of the heterogeneity within any cultural group rather than applying cultural stereotypes

These culturally sensitive approaches support more accurate distinction between cultural differences and autism features, reducing both false positive and false negative assessments.

Rigidity in approach creates risk of missed diagnoses when assessment methods are not appropriately adapted to individual needs and circumstances:

Failing to adapt assessment to individual needs may occur when:

1. Standardized protocols are followed inflexibly despite being poorly suited to the specific individual
2. Communication accommodations are not made for individuals with anxiety, language differences, or processing challenges
3. Sensory needs are not addressed in the assessment environment, creating barriers to accurate evaluation
4. The pace of assessment is not adjusted for individuals with varying processing speeds or attention spans
5. Assessment approaches developed for one population are applied without modification to different groups

This procedural rigidity may create artificial barriers to accurate assessment rather than facilitating genuine understanding of the individual's neurodevelopmental profile.

Person-centred adaptations that maintain assessment validity while accommodating individual needs include:

1. Selection of assessment methods appropriate to the individual's cognitive and communication abilities
2. Environmental modifications addressing sensory sensitivities that might interfere with assessment

3. Flexible pacing allowing processing time and breaks when needed
4. Communication adaptations using the individual's preferred or most effective communication modes
5. Creative approaches to gathering developmental information when standard informant interviews are not possible

These individualized adaptations enhance rather than compromise assessment validity by removing unnecessary barriers to accurate evaluation.

Online assessment considerations deserve special attention, as remote approaches have become increasingly common following the COVID-19 pandemic:

Online experience is significantly better for ASD level 1 (requiring support) compared to levels 2-3 (requiring substantial or very substantial support), creating important distinctions in the appropriateness of remote assessment:

For individuals with ASD level 1 (less severe autism presentations), online assessment offers several advantages:

1. Reduced anxiety in familiar home environment compared to unfamiliar clinical settings
2. Elimination of travel-related stress and sensory challenges
3. Access to assessment despite geographic barriers or mobility limitations
4. Opportunity to observe the individual in their natural environment
5. Greater comfort discussing sensitive topics from personal space

These advantages make online assessment a potentially appropriate option for many adults with less severe autism presentations, particularly those with good verbal abilities and technology access.

However, for ASD levels 2-3 (more severe autism presentations), face-to-face interaction often remains essential because:

1. Communication limitations may make remote interaction difficult or impossible
2. Support needs during assessment may require physical presence
3. Observation of motor mannerisms and physical behaviour's is limited by camera frame
4. Complex sensory assessment requires direct observation
5. Significant cognitive or attention difficulties may interfere with technology engagement

These limitations make remote assessment generally inappropriate as the primary approach for individuals with more substantial support needs, though hybrid models incorporating some remote elements may still be beneficial.

When implementing online assessment for appropriate candidates, important considerations include:

1. Pre-assessment technology checks and support to ensure successful connection
2. Modified administration procedures for standardized instruments, following publisher guidelines for remote use
3. Greater reliance on questionnaires and rating scales completed in advance
4. Creative approaches to observational assessment using structured activities visible on camera
5. Involvement of support persons to assist with technology and assessment activities when needed

These adaptations help maximize the effectiveness of online assessment while recognizing its inherent limitations compared to in-person evaluation.

By recognizing these common pitfalls and implementing strategies to avoid or address them, clinicians can significantly enhance the quality and accuracy of adult autism assessment. This awareness supports more sophisticated clinical practice that adapts to the complex and varied presentations of autism in adulthood while maintaining necessary diagnostic rigor.

CHAPTER 44

Communicating with Autistic Adults

Effective communication with autistic adults during the assessment process is essential for gathering accurate information, building rapport, and ensuring a positive and productive assessment experience. Understanding and accommodating autism-specific communication preferences and needs demonstrates respect while enhancing the quality of the assessment. Adapting communication approaches recognizes that traditional clinical interviewing methods may create unnecessary barriers for many autistic individuals and that simple modifications can significantly improve both the experience and outcomes of assessment.

Clear language that is concrete, specific, and unambiguous helps prevent misunderstandings and reduces cognitive load during assessment interactions:

Concrete language using specific examples rather than abstract concepts supports more accurate communication. For example:

1. Instead of asking "*How is your social life?*" ask "*Who do you spend time with outside of work or school?*"
2. Rather than exploring "communication difficulties," ask about specific situations like "*What happens when you're in a group conversation with several people talking?*"
3. Instead of discussing "sensory sensitivities" generally, ask "*Are there specific sounds, lights, or textures that bother you more than they seem to bother other people?*"
4. Rather than asking about "special interests," inquire "*What topics or activities do you enjoy spending time on, learning about, or collecting?*"
5. Instead of abstract questions about emotions, ask about physical sensations and thoughts associated with specific situations

This concrete approach reduces the interpretive demands of communication and helps ensure that both parties are discussing the same concepts.

Specific language avoids ambiguity that might be difficult for literal interpretation:

1. Instead of "*Could you tell me about your childhood?*" (which could be answered simply "Yes"), ask "*Please describe your experiences in primary school, including friendships and any difficulties you remember*"
2. Rather than "*How do you find social situations?*" (which could be interpreted as asking how to locate them), ask "*What is your experience in social gatherings with unfamiliar people?*"
3. Instead of idioms like "keeping in touch with friends," use precise language like *"How often do you communicate with friends, and how do you do this?"*
4. Rather than asking if something happens "a lot" (which is subjective), ask "*How many times per day/week does this happen?*"
5. Instead of vague quantifiers like "sometimes" or "often," provide specific frequency options like "daily," "weekly," or "monthly"

This precision reduces the need to interpret intended meaning beyond the literal words, which can be challenging for many autistic individuals.

Unambiguous questions with single rather than multiple elements help prevent confusion:

1. Ask one question at a time rather than compound questions that address multiple points
2. Clearly indicate when changing topics rather than making abrupt transitions
3. Specify the type of answer being sought (e.g., "Please describe in a few sentences..." or "A yes or no answer is fine here")
4. Provide context for why information is being requested to clarify its relevance
5. Offer response options when appropriate to clarify the expected type of answer

This structured approach to questioning reduces processing demands and helps ensure that both questions and answers are clearly understood.

Processing time is essential for many autistic individuals to fully comprehend questions, formulate responses, and regulate their communication:

Allowing time to process questions without rushing or interrupting supports more thoughtful and accurate responses:

1. Pause after asking questions rather than immediately rephrasing or prompting
2. Become comfortable with longer silences than might be typical in neurotypical conversation

3. Offer reassurance that taking time to think is perfectly acceptable
4. Watch for signs that the person is still processing rather than assuming they're finished
5. Consider offering the option to write responses for complex questions

This patience with processing time acknowledges the different information processing patterns common in autism and prevents the anxiety and rushed responses that often result from time pressure.

Extended time for complex topics may be needed beyond typical appointment structures:

1. Schedule longer or additional sessions for particularly complex assessment components
2. Offer breaks during longer discussions to allow processing and recovery time
3. Consider splitting assessment components across multiple shorter sessions rather than fewer longer ones
4. Provide preview information before sessions so processing can begin in advance
5. Allow time for processing between sessions rather than scheduling appointments too close together

This flexible approach to timing recognizes that processing complex social and emotional information may require significantly more cognitive effort and time for autistic individuals.

Written information before or during sessions can support verbal processing:

1. Provide written questions in advance of appointments for preview and preparation
2. Offer the option to respond in writing to particularly complex or emotional questions
3. Use visual timelines, diagrams, or other supports during history-taking
4. Provide note-taking materials or allow typing during sessions
5. Follow up verbal sessions with written summaries of key points discussed

These written supports recognize that many autistic individuals process written information more effectively than verbal information, particularly for complex or emotional content.

Alternative formats for communication may be preferred by some individuals and should be offered when possible:

1. Email or text-based communication for certain assessment components
2. Drawing or diagramming options for expressing complex experiences
3. Rating scales or visual analogy scales for quantifying subjective experiences
4. Communication through shared activities rather than direct face-to-face conversation

Disclaimer

This training material represents the professional opinions and clinical perspectives of Dr. Sai Achuthan and Dr. Dave Barker, based on their extensive clinical experience and understanding of autism spectrum disorder across diverse cultural contexts. The content reflects their synthesis of current research and clinical practice as of May 2025 but should not be considered as the only approach to autism assessment.

Understanding autism spectrum disorder requires lifelong learning and continuous engagement with evolving research across different continental perspectives. Cultural, geographical, and individual differences significantly impact how autism manifests and is understood. This training material attempts to address these variations while acknowledging that all clinical approaches contain inherent biases and limitations that must be recognized.

The authors and any organizations they represent cannot be held legally responsible for clinical decisions made based on this training material. All clinical judgments should integrate this information with professional standards, local guidelines, up-to-date research, and the unique needs of each individual being assessed. Clinical practice should always prioritize the wellbeing of the individual being assessed over rigid adherence to any specific assessment framework.

All information presented has been referenced where possible to provide evidence-based foundation for the assessment approaches described. However, clinical judgment remains essential when applying these principles to specific cases, and practitioners should maintain awareness of the evolving nature of autism research and practice.

This material is intended for educational purposes for qualified healthcare professionals and should be used to complement, not replace, comprehensive clinical training and supervision in autism assessment.

Glossary

ABAS-3 - Adaptive Behaviour Assessment System, Third Edition. A standardized measure of adaptive skills across conceptual, social, and practical domains.

ADI-R - Autism Diagnostic Interview-Revised. A comprehensive structured interview for obtaining developmental history from parents or caregivers, considered a gold standard in autism assessment.

ADOS-2 - Autism Diagnostic Observation Schedule, Second Edition. The gold standard observational assessment tool for autism spectrum disorder across the lifespan.

Alexithymia - Difficulty identifying and describing emotions, commonly associated with autism.

AQ - Autism Spectrum Quotient. A self-report screening measure assessing autistic traits across five domains.

ARFID - Avoidant/Restrictive Food Intake Disorder. An eating disorder that may co-occur with autism due to sensory sensitivities.

ASD - Autism Spectrum Disorder. The current diagnostic term encompassing the range of autism presentations.

Camouflaging - Conscious or unconscious strategies used to hide or compensate for autism features in social situations.

Central Coherence - The cognitive tendency to process information in context for global meaning; often described as 'weak' in autism.

Comorbidity - The presence of one or more additional conditions co-occurring with a primary condition.

DCD - Developmental Coordination Disorder. A condition affecting motor coordination that frequently co-occurs with autism.

DSM-5-TR - Diagnostic and Statistical Manual of Mental Disorders, Fifth Edition, Text Revision. The American psychiatric diagnostic manual.

Echolalia - Repetition of words or phrases, which can be immediate or delayed, often seen in autism.

Executive Function - Cognitive processes including planning, working memory, attention, problem-solving, and mental flexibility.

ICD-11 - International Classification of Diseases, 11th Edition. The World Health Organization's diagnostic classification system used in the UK.

Interoception - The perception of internal bodily sensations such as hunger, thirst, or heartbeat.

Masking - The deliberate suppression of behaviours that might appear unusual, particularly repetitive movements or stimming.

NICE - National Institute for Health and Care Excellence. UK organization providing evidence-based healthcare guidelines.

Neurodiversity - The concept that neurological differences like autism are natural variations in human neurology rather than deficits.

Neurotypical - Individuals whose neurological development and functioning are typical of the majority population.

PDD-NOS - Pervasive Developmental Disorder-Not Otherwise Specified. A former diagnostic category now subsumed under ASD.

Proprioception - The sense of body position and movement in space.

RAADS-R - Ritvo Autism Asperger Diagnostic Scale-Revised. A self-report measure designed for diagnosing autism in adults.

RRBs - Restricted and Repetitive Behaviours. One of the two core diagnostic domains of autism.

SAD - Social Anxiety Disorder. A condition that may co-occur with or be mistaken for autism.

SCD - Social (Pragmatic) Communication Disorder. A condition involving social communication difficulties without restricted/repetitive behaviours.

Sensory Processing - How the nervous system receives, organizes, and responds to sensory information.

SPD - Sensory Processing Disorder. Difficulties with sensory processing that may occur independently or as part of autism.

SRS-2 - Social Responsiveness Scale-2. An observer-rated measure of social impairment associated with autism.

Stimming - Self-stimulatory behaviours such as hand-flapping, rocking, or spinning, often serving sensory or regulatory functions.

Theory of Mind - The ability to understand that others have thoughts, feelings, and perspectives different from one's own.

WAIS-IV - Wechsler Adult Intelligence Scale, Fourth Edition. The most widely used intelligence test for adults.

WHODAS 2.0 - World Health Organization Disability Assessment Schedule. A standardized measure of health and disability across cultures.

Appendix Content

Appendix A: Assessment Tools Quick Reference Guide

Screening Measures:

- **Autism Spectrum Quotient (AQ) - 50 items, self-report**
- AQ-10 - Brief screening version
- RAADS-R - 80 items, includes developmental dimension

Diagnostic Instruments:

- ADOS-2 Module 4 - For verbally fluent adolescents and adults
- ADI-R - Developmental history interview
- 3Di - Computerized alternative to ADI-R

Functional Measures:

- WHODAS 2.0 - Global disability assessment
- Vineland-3 - Adaptive behaviour scales
- ABAS-3 - Adaptive functioning across domains

Supplementary Measures:

- SRS-2 - Social responsiveness (observer-rated)
- Sensory Profile (Adult version)
- Reading the Mind in the Eyes Test
- Executive function questionnaires (e.g., BRIEF-A)

Appendix B: ICD-11 Diagnostic Codes for Autism Spectrum Disorder

- **6A02.0** - ASD without disorder of intellectual development and with mild or no impairment of functional language
- **6A02.1** - ASD with disorder of intellectual development and with mild or no impairment of functional language

- **6A02.2** - ASD without disorder of intellectual development and with impaired functional language
- **6A02.3** - ASD with disorder of intellectual development and with impaired functional language
- **6A02.4** - ASD without disorder of intellectual development and with absence of functional language
- **6A02.5** - ASD with disorder of intellectual development and with absence of functional language
- **6A02.Y** - Other specified autism spectrum disorder
- **6A02.Z** - Autism Spectrum Disorder, unspecified

Appendix C: Sample Assessment Report Template

[Insight Diagnostics Global Limited]

AUTISM SPECTRUM DISORDER ASSESSMENT REPORT

Patient Details:

- Name:
- NHS Number:
- Date of Birth:
- Assessment Dates:
- Report Date:

1. Referral Information

- Source of referral
- Reason for referral
- Background information

2. Assessment Methods

- Clinical interviews conducted
- Standardized instruments administered
- Collateral information sources
- Documents reviewed

3. Developmental History

- Early development
- Educational history
- Employment history

- Relationship history
- Medical history

4. Current Presentation

- Social communication and interaction
- Restricted and repetitive behaviours
- Sensory sensitivities
- Cognitive and language abilities
- Mental health
- Functional impact

5. Assessment Results

- Standardized test results
- Observational findings
- Collateral information

6. Formulation

- Integration of findings
- Developmental trajectory
- Strengths and challenges

7. Diagnosis

- Diagnostic conclusion
- ICD-11 classification
- Co-occurring conditions
- Differential diagnosis considered

8. Recommendations

- Immediate support needs
- Long-term interventions
- Environmental modifications
- Further assessments
- Resources and services

Clinician Signature: Date: Sai Achuthan

Appendix D: Resources for Autistic Adults in the UK

National Organizations:

□ National Autistic Society: www.autism.org.uk

□ Autistica: www.autistica.org.uk

□ Ambitious about Autism: www.ambitiousaboutautism.org.uk

□ Autism Alliance: www.autism-alliance.org.uk

Government Resources:

□ Access to Work: www.gov.uk/access-to-work

□ Equality and Human Rights Commission: www.equalityhumanrights.com

Online Communities:

□ Autistic UK: www.autisticuk.org

□ ARGH (Autistic Rights Group Highland)

□ Various regional autism support groups

Employment Support:

□ National Autistic Society Employment Services

□ Specialisterne UK

□ Autism Plus Employment Services

Benefits Information:

□ Personal Independence Payment (PIP)

□ Employment and Support Allowance (ESA)

□ Disabled Students' Allowance (DSA)

Appendix E: Cultural Considerations Checklist

Pre-Assessment:

□ Identify client's cultural background

□ Arrange culturally appropriate interpreter if needed

□ Review cultural norms for social communication

□ Consider religious/spiritual factors

□ Plan culturally sensitive assessment approaches

During Assessment:

- ☐ Adapt eye contact expectations
- ☐ Consider cultural communication patterns
- ☐ Adjust personal space norms
- ☐ Recognize cultural emotion expression
- ☐ Account for family structure variations

Post-Assessment:

- ☐ Frame diagnosis culturally appropriately
- ☐ Provide culturally relevant resources
- ☐ Consider cultural stigma factors
- ☐ Adapt recommendations to cultural context
- ☐ Engage community supports

Reference

Antshel, K. M., & Russo, N. (2019). Autism spectrum disorders and ADHD: Overlapping phenomenology, diagnostic issues, and treatment considerations. *Current Psychiatry Reports, 21(5), 34.*

Antshel, K. M., Zhang-James, Y., Wagner, K. E., Ledesma, A., & Faraone, S. V. (2016). An update on the comorbidity of ADHD and ASD: A focus on clinical management. *Expert review of neurotherapeutics, 16(3), 279-293.*

Brown, L., & Memmott, J. (2013). The role of document design in enhancing accessibility of clinical reports. *Journal of Clinical Documentation, 28(2), 34-41.*

Carpenter, P. (2012). Diagnostic decision-making in autism assessment. Journal of Developmental Disorders, 15(3), 78-89.

Crane, L., Chester, J. W., Goddard, L., Henry, L. A., & Hill, E. (2018). Experiences of autism diagnosis: A survey of over 1000 parents in the United Kingdom. Autism, 22(4), 70-81.

Demetriou, E. A., Lampit, A., Quintana, D. S., Naismith, S. L., Song, Y. J. C., Pye, J. E., Hickie, I., & Guastella, A. J. (2018). Autism spectrum disorders: A meta-analysis of executive function. *Molecular Psychiatry, 23(5), 1198-1204.*

Gernsbacher, M. A., Raimond, A. R., Balinghasay, M. T., & Boston, J. S. (2016). "Special needs" is an ineffective euphemism. *Cognitive Research: Principles and Implications, 1(1), 113-120.*

Geurts, H. M., Luman, M., & Van Meel, C. S. (2009). What's in a game: The effect of social motivation on interference control in boys with ADHD and autism spectrum disorders. Journal of Child Psychology and Psychiatry, 50(6), 672-681.

Goldman, S., Wang, C., Salgado, M. W., Greene, P. E., Kim, M., & Rapin, I. (2009). Motor stereotypies in children with autism and other developmental disorders. *Developmental Medicine & Child Neurology, 51(1), 30-38.*

Howlin, P., & Moss, P. (2012). Adults with autism spectrum disorders. *The Canadian Journal of Psychiatry, 57(5), 275-283.*

Jones, R. S., Huws, J. C., & Beck, G. (2015). Enhancing accessibility in autism diagnostic reports. Good Autism Practice, 16(1), 185-192.

Kenny, L., Hattersley, C., Molins, B., Buckley, C., Povey, C., & Pellicano, E. (2016). Which terms should be used to describe autism? Perspectives from the UK autism community. *Autism, 20(4), 442-462.*

Lai, M. C., Kassee, C., Besney, R., Bonato, S., Hull, L., Mandy, W., Szatmari, P., & Ameis, S. H. (2019). Prevalence of co-occurring mental health diagnoses in the autism population: A systematic review and meta-analysis. *The Lancet Psychiatry, 6(10), 819-829.*

Leekam, S. R., Libby, S. J., Wing, L., Gould, J., & Taylor, C. (2015). The Diagnostic Interview for Social and Communication Disorders: Algorithms for ICD-10 childhood autism and Wing and Gould autistic spectrum disorder. Journal of Child Psychology and Psychiatry, 43(3), 50-61.

Lewis, L. F. (2016). Exploring the experience of self-diagnosis of autism spectrum disorder in adults. *Archives of Psychiatric Nursing, 30(5), 575-580.*

Lichtenstein, P., Carlström, E., Råstam, M., Gillberg, C., & Anckarsäter, H. (2010). The genetics of autism spectrum disorders and related neuropsychiatric disorders in childhood. *American Journal of Psychiatry, 167(11), 1357-1363.*

Little, L. M., Dean, E., Tomchek, S. D., & Dunn, W. (2018). Sensory processing patterns in autism, attention deficit hyperactivity disorder, and typical development. *Physical & Occupational Therapy in Pediatrics, 38(3), 243-254.*

Lord, C., Elsabbagh, M., Baird, G., & Veenstra-Vanderweele, J. (2018). Autism spectrum disorder. *The Lancet, 392(10146), 508-520.*

Mahajan, R., Bernal, M. P., Panzer, R., Whitaker, A., Roberts, W., Handen, B., Hardan, A., Anagnostou, E., & Veenstra-VanderWeele, J. (2012). Clinical practice pathways for evaluation and medication choice for attention-deficit/hyperactivity disorder symptoms in autism spectrum disorders. *Pediatrics, 130(Supplement_2), S125-S138.*

Mandy, W., & Lai, M. C. (2016). Annual Research Review: The role of the environment in the developmental psychopathology of autism spectrum condition. *Journal of Child Psychology and Psychiatry, 57(3), 271-292.*

Milton, D., & Bracher, M. (2013). Autistics speak but are they heard. *Medical Sociology Online, 7(2), 61-69.*

Ne'eman, A., & Kapp, S. (2012). What are the stakes? An analysis of the impact of the neurodiversity movement on policy and practice. In J. Davidson & M. Orsini (Eds.), Worlds of Autism (pp. 62-75). University of Minnesota Press.

Nicolaidis, C., Raymaker, D., McDonald, K., Dern, S., Ashkenazy, E., Boisclair, C., Robertson, S., & Baggs, A. (2014). Participatory research with autistic communities: Shifting the system. In S. Htz (Ed.), Autism in Translation (pp. 135-152). Palgrave Macmillan.

Nijmeijer, J. S., Minderaa, R. B., Buitelaar, J. K., Mulligan, A., Hartman, C. A., & Hoekstra, P. J. (2008). Attention-deficit/hyperactivity disorder and social dysfunctioning. *Clinical Psychology Review, 28(4), 692-708.*

Rommelse, N. N., Franke, B., Geurts, H. M., Hartman, C. A., & Buitelaar, J. K. (2017). Shared heritability of attention-deficit/hyperactivity disorder and autism spectrum disorder. European Child & Adolescent Psychiatry, 26(4), 427-438.

Roux, A. M., Shattuck, P. T., Rast, J. E., Rava, J. A., & Anderson, K. A. (2015). National Autism Indicators Report: Transition into Young Adulthood. Life Course Outcomes Research Program, A.J. Drexel Autism Institute, Drexel University.

Rutherford, M., McKenzie, K., Johnson, T., Catchpole, C., O'Hare, A., McClure, I., & Murray, A. (2018). Gender ratio in a clinical population sample, age of diagnosis and duration of assessment in children and adults with autism spectrum disorder. *Autism, 22(1), 119-128.*

Sarrett, J. C., & Kapp, S. K. (2018). Self-identification and self-diagnosis in the autistic community. In R. Hacking & R. Yergeau (Eds.), Authoring Autism (pp. 85-104). Duke University Press.

Taylor, L. J., Eapen, V., Maybery, M. T., Midford, S., Paynter, J., Quarmby, L., Smith, T., Williams, K., & Whitehouse, A. J. (2016). Diagnostic evaluation for autism spectrum disorder: A survey of health professionals in Australia. *BMJ Open, 6(9), e012517.*

Taylor, M., & Marrable, T. (2011). Access to social care for adults with autism spectrum conditions. School for Social Care Research, London School of Economics and Political Science.

INSIGHT
DIAGNOSTICS
GLOBAL

www.ingramcontent.com/pod-product-compliance
Ingram Content Group UK Ltd.
Pitfield, Milton Keynes, MK11 3LW, UK
UKHW060058200726
13845UKWH00048B/141

9 789371 393522